To Carolina,
A Wonderfully-Sweet Person.
Yours in great health!
Cheers!
Chef Peter

MW01109472

Better Food for A Better You

Better Food for A Better You

Peter Klarman

ISBN 978-1-300-06551-7

Disclosure:

The author of this book does not dispense medical advice or prescribe the use of any technique as a form of treatment for physical, emotional, or medical problems without the advice of a physician, either directly or indirectly. The intent of the author is only to offer information of a general nature to help you in your quest for better eating habits. In the event you use any of the information in this book for yourself, the author and the publisher assume no responsibility for your actions.

For Aunt Betty

Oh, Thank You's!

This book would not have been possible without the patience, care, love, and support of the following individuals:

To my family: Thanks to my Mom for always loving and supporting me, my Aunt Betty for her deep wisdom and open-ears, my older brothers Mike and Howie for gladly testing and critiquing my recipes, and to the rest of my extended family for all the Sunday family gatherings.

To my Dad: Thank you for raising me, your courage in facing your illness, and for the lessons you taught me in life and in death.

To Mike Bernier, my mentor, and friend: thank you for the sagely advice, friendship, and your many *metaphorical* kicks in the ass to help me stay on track.

To all of the great music makers, thanks to my musical friends: Paul and Grace Dell Aquila, Billy 'Rock' Rayner, Greg Hauser, Davey G., Matt Gallager, Pete Petersen, Danny Kiely, Pauly Zarb, Chris Bradley, Rafael Barake & Astrid Gonzalez, Diego Palma, Doug Florio & Kimmet Cantwell, Dom Famularo (my inspirational, musical mentor), all the incredible drummers, and musicians that continue inspiring me to play.

To my culinary friends and peers, thank you for all the gastronomic inspiration: Anita Steineck, Christopher Seckham, Roxanne Koteles Smith, Coco Tran, Dorit D., the Rappa brothers, Tim Tucker, Marcus Wilkerson, and Mark Williams.

To the health practitioners who helped me improve in some way along the way and were so patient with my impatience, huge thanks go out to Jeff LaGree, Christopher Skeen, Wayne Goodlet, Tyler and Cindy Richmond, Bill Parravano, Harry Gallager, James O'dell, Janet Clarke, Monika Grille, Ted and Lillian Hollinger, Karen Kremer, and Marilyn Whittenberg.

Thanks to all of the creative people that helped me in finishing this book: Cindy Davis for her wonderfully delicious photography, Eric DeYoung for his foreword, critical thinking, wisdom, and guidance.

Very special thanks go out to Amanda L. LeDuke for her spot-on editing skills, hard work, critiquing recipes, and patience while keeping me from straying too far from the real story. And thank you to Mr. Frodo, Cooper, Jonah P., and Cheeky for being such very nice boys.

Other special thanks go out to my good friend Iman Ali for his technical assistance, support, and many creative ideas, Summer and the staff at Rainbow Blossom for their continued support, all my former co-workers from the late great Wild Oats (R.I.P.), Nate Peterson and Carole Bretschneider and the crew from Earthsave for their cheerleading and pure inspiration, Angelina W. for loving all of the raw pizzas, Chase Barmore of Life Bar Louisville, Rehmannia Dean Thomas for sharing his remarkable herbal wisdom, my chef mentor Tim Tucker and The Salvation Army Center of Hope Culinary training program, Gary Null for the provocative insights on health and nutrition he shares in every show, Robert O. Young for his ground-breaking work in microbiology, biochemistry, and microscopy, Shelley R. Young for her innovative, delicious, and alkalizing cuisine, David Wolfe for his health conscious enthusiasm, and thanks to all the great chefs and authors that inspired me to create *Better Food for a Better You.*

Table of Contents:

Enchanting Entrees

Delightful Desserts

Foreword
Dr. Eric DeYoung

According to the World Health Organization; "The U. S. spends a higher portion of its gross domestic product on health than any other country but ranks 37 out of 191 countries according to its performance." WHO Director-General Dr. Gro Harlem Brundtland says: "The main message from this report is that the health and well-being of people around the world depend critically on the performance of the health systems that serve them. Yet there is wide variation in performance, even among countries with similar levels of income and health expenditure. It is essential for decision-makers to understand the underlying reasons so that system performance, and hence the health of populations, can be improved."

Dr. Christopher Murray, Director of WHO's Global Programme on Evidence for Health Policy says: "Although significant progress has been achieved in past decades, virtually all countries are underutilizing the resources that are available to them. This leads to large numbers of preventable deaths and disabilities; unnecessary suffering, injustice, inequality and denial of an individual's basic rights to health."

As a Doctor of Traditional Naturopathy and Occupational Therapist, clients come to my practice when the conventional medical model hasn't improved their level of health, didn't offer them solutions to their conditions, or in some cases actually caused them more harm than good. These are unfortunate truths for many in the United States and even in other countries. Clients are intuitively seeking solutions for their state of health and ultimately not seeking medication or surgery as their only options. Far too often the conventional medical model teaches "Feel Better" as their motto towards "health and wellness." Simply feeling better is the attempt at touching only the tip of the proverbial iceberg. The tip is only on the surface, the majority of the mass of one's health is below the surface and beyond the symptoms. Conventional medicine, as a philosophy and business, attempts to treat the immediate symptoms which are absolutely necessary in an acute urgent situation where life and death are literally in the hands of the physician. "Feeling better" implies that you have achieved baseline health. When your symptoms are reduced, masked, or suppressed you should "feel better." However, the root cause of your symptoms occurring in the first place may not have been dealt with and often clients have no direction or plan or even understanding as to why they had symptoms of ill health to begin with. The base of the iceberg has not been addressed leaving still a mass of ill health choices, behaviors, and conditions unaddressed.

True wellness, on the other hand, is based on the idea that one's health is more complex, involves greater awareness, education, responsibility, and assistance in order to help the client achieve independence from the conventional medical model. Clients should seek advice and clarity in supporting health without medication management. Natural health practitioners need to empower the client to assume responsibility for their health choices and encourage them not to be dependent on a healthcare provider dictating and telling them what they must do for their health. For chronically ill clients with years of metabolic distress and unresolved pathology, our model must adapt to include true prevention and true wellness. A quick fix hasn't worked and more pharmaceutical treatments haven't been the solution when, as a society, the United States consumes the most but is still 37th in the world.

In my professional opinion, the basic difference between true wellness and the standard practice of symptom management lies in the practitioners' knowledge and experience in nutrition-based medicine. Having treated tens of thousands of clients with chronic medical diagnoses there are common denominators shared by the majority, that common connection is lack of knowledge and appreciation for true nutrition. This is appreciated in many medical articles and journal discussions.

"Nutrition plays a critical role in numerous pathophysiological conditions, including such prevalent diseases as diabetes, cancer, and cardiovascular disease. Despite the recognition that physicians are often called upon to provide guidance in nutritional aspects of disease and disease prevention, nutrition has not been consistently emphasized in medical school curricula. Indeed, numerous reports suggest that nutrition education of physicians remains inadequate. A 1997-1998 analysis of data provided by the Clinical Administrative Data Service of the Association of American Medical Colleges (AAMC) found that only 33 accredited U.S. medical schools (26%) had a required nutrition course *[An average of 18 ± 12 hours of nutrition was required, including material integrated into other types of courses.]* Other reports on the status of nutrition in medical education have presented a similar picture. Over the years, such reports have led to frequent calls for increased emphasis on, and reform of, nutrition education of physicians." (Survey of Nutrition Education in U.S. Medical Schools – An Instructor-Based

Analysis; Frank M. Torti, Jr., Kelly M. Adams, MPH, RD, Lloyd J. Edwards, PhD, Karen C. Lindell, MS, RD, Steven H. Zeisel, MD, PhD)

Nutrition is the critical link to true health and true wellness in this country and around the world. As a society we must engage in improving the quality of food choices made available to us in our grocery stores, our children's cafeterias and in our local restaurants. We are over- consuming empty calorie foods, Genetically Modified (GMO) foods, processed, overheated, packaged, container, and fast foods which are filled with toxins, poisons, hormones, antibiotics, vaccines and other synthetic and harmful ingredients which affect your health, your child's health and the health of developing fetuses. This compromises our welfare and amplifies our need for proper medical management.

"Recent research shows 45 percent of high-fructose corn syrup in commercial food products contains mercury, a known toxin," Dr. Anne Kelly (former faculty member in general pediatrics at the University of Minnesota) told a group of medical professionals in Peoria (2010). "We have an estimated 10,000 new chemicals in the environment and no idea what the effect is on children," she said. "With this multitude of chemicals, the reality is we don't know what we're dealing with." In 2009, two U.S. studies found that nearly half of tested samples of commercial high-fructose corn syrup contained mercury. On average, American adults consume about 12 teaspoons daily of high-fructose corn syrup, but teens and other high consumers take in up to 80 percent more than that. "Mercury is toxic in all its forms. Given how much high-fructose corn syrup is consumed by children, it could be an additional source of mercury never before considered," Dr. David Wallinga, a co-author of both studies of this issue with the Institute for Agriculture and Trade Policy.

High-fructose corn syrup is just one of many examples of food contamination and environmental toxins. Ever heard the statement "you are what you eat"? There is a great deal of truth to this statement. Now if you eat a chicken you are not going to turn into a chicken. But what the chicken was raised on will be ingested by you when you eat it. As long as farmers are allowed to spray environmental toxins on the food they produce, they will be poisoning you and your family along with the insects they are trying to kill. These pesticides are in the actual flesh of the produce, carried by the winds far from the field where they were originally sprayed; they are in the soil, in the groundwater, in the fish that swim in the water and in the animals that eat the feed that were sprayed and consumed by your body.

Children are also more sensitive to environmental toxins than adults, so the damage from environmental toxins often manifests sooner in babies and children.

According to the National Cancer Institute, cancer incidence among children under the age of 15 increased 32 percent between 1950 and 1985. It has also been estimated by researchers that there is a large percentage of cancer occurrences caused by exposure to environmental toxins found in our food supply. It is overwhelming trying to capture all the news, research, updates, journal articles, marketing ads, etc. It is time that the people of the United States take a stand for true health and true wellness by educating yourself about health, nutrition, proper supplementation, healthy clean food and water, and be empowered to discuss this with your physician. You might be the only real source of information and can partner with your healthcare provider in ensuring you go from "feeling better to being well."

That being said, we have an opportunity to make great changes in our healthcare delivery system, in the recommendations and choices available to clients, and to properly educate our healthcare providers about true nutrition and wellness. As a consumer you too have choices to make. Instead of driving through the fast food line why not consider packing your lunch with food from your home garden, stopping for a sit down meal and choosing healthy/lite meals or going to the grocery store and buying something fresh to eat. Instead of buying a soft drink consider filtered water or a veggie juice drink, a real fruit smoothie or some herbal tea. Next time you go out with your family to eat, use the time to educate your children about healthy food choices. If you make meal times educational you are more likely to make healthier choices and you encourage your children to make good choices too. Choose side items where most of the fruits and vegetables are located, salads and soups and consider sharing entrees to control portions, conserve costs, and reduce waste. By asking for filtered water when you are out to eat you can save about $2.50 per drink by not buying tea and soft drinks.

Be conscious about the foods you eat. Consider that everything you put in your body is supposed to give you proper fuel, energy, vitamins, minerals, and healthy probiotics to support your immune system. Reduce your sugar content from simple sugars (not fruits) and increase your proteins from non-dairy/animal sources like beans, rice, quinoa, seeds, and nuts. Rather than sit on the couch after dinner or run right back to work, go for a walk, take a bike ride, do some sit ups or push-ups. Consider joining a fitness or wellness center as a family, again, encouraging everyone to be responsible for their health habits. If you are constantly around negative, unhealthy people, you might need to move away from them, and resonate around healthier more positive people who will support a healthy lifestyle.

Whether we want to admit it or not, our health is our choice. We can make changes today regardless of what the medical reports suggests, regardless of the

EPA reports, regardless what your parents taught you. You have choices to guide you towards a healthier lifestyle. If you are always thinking about living a healthy lifestyle then you will always be considering healthy choices. It is not alright to blame your family history, your doctor, the pharmacy, or the food industry. You can grow your own foods, buy organic produce, prepare your own meals, and make healthier choices regardless of where you go to eat.

"Let food be thy medicine and medicine be thy food." Stated by Hippocrates centuries ago, we have gone far away from this concept in this country. Chef Peter Klarman in his book, *Better Food for A Better You,* invites you to explore the health value of eating healthy foods. Chef Peter comes from a unique background growing up in a family with adopted belief patterns, poor food choices, and common bad habits leading to his own health imbalances. When you go through a personal experience associated with your health, it molds you to become a resource in how to regain your health. There are lessons to be learned from all experiences in life. Chef Peter's experiences have inspired him to write a book about lifestyle change. This book isn't just about food recipes and special ingredients. It is a book about empowerment, about inspiration, and about encouragement to do something great with your life through healthy living habits and great tasting food. As a fan of healthy foods, I must say that Chef Peter's recipes are fabulous and I invite you to try more of his recommendations at every meal. The flavor of his food and the content of this great book will leave you asking for more, please!

Dr. Eric M. DeYoung is a doctor of traditional naturopathy, an occupational therapist, author, friend, and founder of The Center for Alternative Medicine/Occupational Kinetics in Louisville, Kentucky.

A note to the reader

The purpose of this book is to provide you with tasty recipes, and resources and information on ways to support and nurture the part of you that wants to learn to prepare delicious and healthy foods and make steady progress toward improving your quality of life. The idea is simple. By preparing more of your meals using home-grown, locally-grown, or natural and organically produced foods, the more control you have over the food that goes into your body. The basic idea behind this is to provide the body with the proper nutrition it requires to support your daily health. That's all there is to it. You put together more of your own meals without having to become a professional chef; just your own personal chef. This book provides over 70 easy-to-prepare and delicious recipes to help you get started. The recipes use a wide variety of plant based, whole-foods and spices which help you experiment with flavor, and develop a deeper sense of taste. Use this book as a tool to find better food choices and information, try the recipes, add in some of your own ideas if you wish and have some fun in the process. Remember, the food is what is most important here.

There's another story to this book. If it interests you, I encourage you to dig into my personal narrative about growing up in a big, food-oriented family, dealing with the illness of a parent with cancer, and the journey I took in transforming my own health and becoming a chef. In addition, for your convenience I've included a few checklists of basic kitchen utensils, spices, etc. to help set-up or re-tool your kitchen. Lastly, you may find the listing of web resources and suggested books helpful in locating high quality foods, nutrient dense super-foods, supplements and useful information on health and nutrition to assist you in learning more about healthy living.

In the meantime, I wish each of you well on your journey to feeling great, having a more youthful energy and glow, enjoying many yummy recipes, discovering new flavors or rediscovering old ones, and having a more vital and productive life. There are many options to improving the quality of your life. My hope is that this collection of recipes will serve as a useful and helpful set of tools to help create a better life for you and your loved ones.

Yours in great health and bon appetit!
Chef Peter

Introduction

The need for proper digestion and the absorption of nutrients is vital to our existence. Presently, chronic diseases, namely, digestive disorders are growing at an alarming rate. In the past 20 years, the rates of childhood obesity and diabetes have skyrocketed and the top three causes of chronic disease and death (heart disease, cancer, and stroke) have increased or remained constant in the United States. The combination of all of these diseases is causing a significant strain on our nation's health and economy and we don't seem to be making much progress in prevention. Now more than ever there are many valid scientific studies that have clearly demonstrated how improving one's diet, lowering stress, and regular exercise can benefit the health of the people of this nation and the world. If you search the internet for recent world health rankings, you may be surprised at what you learn about the quality of health in America. According to recent statistics, our country ranks 37th (in the world) in healthcare and number one in how much we spend on it. It's time for us to make better, more informed choices about what we put into our bodies and to take better care of ourselves. However, despite having good intentions, the best technology and diagnostic techniques that modern medicine currently provides, and all the most wonderful New Year's resolutions, somehow life gets in the way and many people are still dealing with the same health challenges a few months or even years later. Why? It must be understood that dis-ease and health are both processes that are related to our daily food choices. The more we are aware of the effects of those choices, the faster we can start the step-by-step process of awareness, changing thoughts, attitudes and beliefs and, finally, actions and habits. Modern day stresses are always going to be there. The better the quality of your daily diet, or rather food lifestyle, the better you will be at handling stress, the more balanced you will be physically, mentally, spiritually, and the better you will be able to respond to the challenges in life.

An unfortunate thing in this society is that many people wait until the quality of their health is so compromised before they do something about it. In many cases, this may mean ending up in an emergency room for costly tests, expensive prescriptions, and huge medical bills. As noted yogi Bikram Choudhury has said, "Your body is your responsibility, you choose!" When you begin to take more responsibility for your own health, you will indeed begin to enjoy the true benefits of a better quality of life and lower medical expenses. It is the goal of this recipe book/food lifestyle transition to help you start or get back on a path to making better food choices and improving the quality of your life. How far you go with it is up to you.

Here are a few questions to ask. How healthy can you be? Have you ever wondered about it or is it something that you never imagined? What's at that end of the scale on the spectrum of health? I believe it's possible to live more happily, energetically, and experience more optimal health. As Chef Shelley Redford Young has said, "nothing tastes as good as good health feels". Vibrant health or chronic disease is not something that you reach one day and just stay there. Each is a result of past and present decisions or actions that are intimately related to daily food choices; choices that are directly under your control. Ultimately, you are the chief caretaker of your mind, body, and spirit on a journey toward health or disease. As humans, the natural state of the body is to be healthy and in balance. However, life and the pressures that come with it seem to get the better of us and results in many of the chronic diseases our society is afflicted with today.

If you wish to dig a little deeper and ask yourself a few more questions, you will find some important clues about the quality of your health. How often do you get sick each year? Do you have any chronic allergies? Do you have any recurring aches and pains? Are you excessively tired every day? Are you addicted to fast food restaurants and junk food each day? Do you smoke or drink alcohol regularly, consume processed packaged foods, and sugary soft drinks? What other chronic stress are you under? How are your relationships with others or yourself? These are just a few important questions to consider.

In order to have a deeper understanding of what good health means it requires you to have more self-knowledge. It's not always easy to understand your own actions and, more importantly, be honest, and open about them. Many of us may have had poor dietary habits, unhealthy lifestyles, suffered from unusually high stress levels, unhealthy relationships, been exposed to countless environmental pollutants, experienced chronic fatigue, aches and pains, and chronic, and acute disease, etc. What lies on the opposite side of living this way? No matter what your current level of health is or why you ended up there, it's time to look more closely at improving the quality of your life. At some point or another in life, you or someone you care about will have to come to terms with a health problem(s) and face the challenge of being responsible for taking care of it.

Whether or not you are currently dealing with health related issues, trying some of the recipes in this book is an opportunity to help enhance your lifestyle in a positive way. This book, or rather recipe coaching guide, provides useful food preparation tips, recipes with ideas for better food substitutions that are simple, do-able, and help assist you in improving or reaching your dietary and lifestyle goals. It contains many easy-to-prepare recipes that have been developed and taste-tested on many of my clients and in cooking classes, and have been created to promote health and well-being. The primary focus of the recipes is on including more whole-food, plant-based, pH balancing foods, and gluten-free dishes that are either minimally-cooked or raw. My hope is to provide appealing recipes that offer delectable flavors, are timely and affordable to prepare, provide a wide variety of foods, and better quality nutrition. The recipes are based on a concept I call "stealth health". Basically, the wide variety of ingredients contained in the recipes help supply you with the vital macronutrients and especially, the micronutrients and phytonutrients (the biologically active, health promoting compounds found mainly in plants) the body needs to allow for proper healing, balance the pH level, and help support health at the cellular level.

Starting out, the task of creating delicious and healthy recipes to help balance the body's pH presented new challenges and required a different way of thinking. The idea I wanted to investigate was this: in order to improve the quality of health and thrive, the body has certain nutritional requirements to be met each day. This book offers you recipes with a wide variety of nutrient-dense foods that assist in fulfilling those needs.

A question arose: by offering a collection of recipes that use more plant-based, whole food, and gluten-free foods as substitutions, how could I create more delicious, satisfying, and health-promoting recipes? The original concept of this book was very similar to the basic idea stated in a song by The Who called 'Substitute.' Is there a better or healthier substitute for an ingredient in any given recipe? Well, the answer is yes, in most cases. At first, the idea sounded nearly impossible or even ridiculous. As many have said, necessity is the mother of invention. This book is the culmination of the following: researching information on food and nutrition, the knowledge and experience gained through having had an illness, and applying some foundational nutritional concepts as a chef to build recipes for those seeking more delicious and healthy options.

Although optimal nutrition was my main concern when I began writing recipes, I realized that optimal nutrition was not necessarily what most people are looking for every day. In my experience as a private chef and working with people, I have learned a lot about the numerous and complex variety of tastes, texture, food and odor sensitivities, and satiety preferences people have. With that in mind, I set out to create recipes that would attempt to meet the following demanding criteria: great tasting, pleasantly aromatic, appealing texture, filling and satisfying, budget friendly, easy to follow and prepare, and promoting of health and longevity.

In addition, the recipes include approximate preparation times. Some take up to fifteen minutes or less, some up to thirty minutes, and others that require up to an hour or more. There are also some tips on how to shorten preparation times. In other words, for any given recipe, you do not have to spend too much of your life stuck in the kitchen!

Lastly, some possible benefits you will encounter by trying the enclosed recipes include: more energy, a well-balanced immune system, hormonal balance, beautiful supple skin and a more youthful appearance, better sleep quality, maintaining your ideal weight while not feeling like you're always counting calories, more sizzle to your love life, and enhanced longevity. You'll also enjoy learning some basic nutritional information about key foods in the recipes, making your health a priority by improving daily food choices, and, if you are running out of meal ideas, have a wider variety of health-promoting recipes available that encourage you take better care of yourself or your family. With an improved quality of life, you can go out and share the wealth of healthy wisdom you have acquired to help grow a better, more sustainable health standard in the community and the world.

Part I
My Story

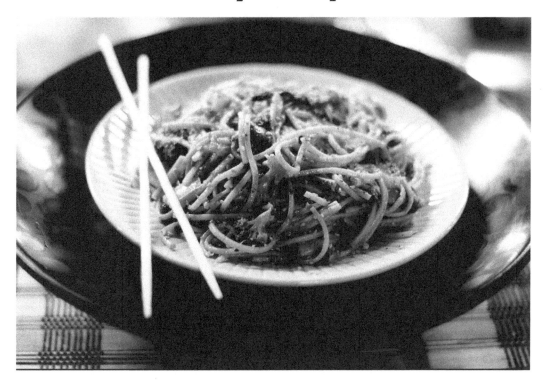

Hello, how are you? Let's eat!

As a youngster from New York growing up in a large family, food was of utmost importance; especially when the families would get together for a big Sunday brunch or a festive holiday dinner. When we arrived at the door for a family gathering, there was always a certain urgency to begin the meal, and that usually began with my aunt or uncle saying, "Hello, how are you? Now that you're here, let's eat!" There was little or no formality to the family meal. The table was set, the food was ready, and everyone was hungry for some eats.

The following describes a typical Sunday brunch and a dinner visit with the families. For the Sunday brunches, there was a smorgasbord of fresh bakery rolls, bagels, bialys, various breads, muffins, and spreads like: butter, various cream cheeses, egg salad, and smoked salmon. The beverages included orange juice, apple juice, regular and diet sodas, coffee, and tea. Finally, for dessert, there was some kind of crumb cake, chocolate layer cake, apple pie, or some fresh fruit salad. After the big brunch, we often settled down in the den to watch the big game.

For the family dinner, we routinely started with a few varieties of fresh bread or rolls, a simple iceberg lettuce or mixed green salad with tomatoes, red cabbage, and shredded carrots topped with various bottled salad dressings. Inevitably, for the entrée, and the largest portion on the plate, there was of some type of cooked beef or poultry on the menu. Grilled hamburgers on a bun, grilled or roasted chicken, steak, ribs, turkey burgers, cured deli meats, and grilled frankfurters were just some of the usual offerings. I grew up in a Jewish family so it was a necessity for all meats and poultry to be certified kosher. For vegetable selections, there were baked or mashed potatoes, potato salad or coleslaw, canned or steamed green beans, fresh grilled corn on the cob, the occasional baked sweet potatoes, and sometimes, french-fried potatoes (a big family favorite).

During the meal, it seemed like the race was on to see which person could finish their plate first. At the time, it was quite amusing, and my cousins and I had competitions to see who could consume the most food. Since I occasionally came in first, I was given the nickname "pound-for-pound" (a silly expression we made up for the ability to eat one's own weight in food). After dinner, everyone was sporting a full belly, and we moved into the den or living room for some more family banter.

When we were in our early teens, my older brothers, cousins, and I used to go outside and play with whatever ball was around or play Frisbee with one of our dogs. However, as we got older, we lost interest in such things and preferred lounging in any room with a TV. One reason for that was there was yet another cherished meal waiting: dessert. Typically, it consisted of a variety of the following: apple pie (a la mode), crumb cake, cheese cake, Neapolitan ice cream, various pastries and cookies, fresh cut melons or fruit salad, watermelon, and freshly brewed coffee or tea. After an abundance of dessert, there was typically one thing left to do, and that was to find the best place to sit or lay down for a while. At this point, we were quite full and tired. Interestingly, after the meal, it often looked like some of the older family members needed help getting up from their chairs. In fact, before the invention of the TV remote, I was appointed the role of the human channel changer. Unfortunately, being the youngest person in the room, I had no say in the matter. Even after the invention of the remote, I was usually the one put in charge of finding it after it was misplaced. Finally after a few hours of TV, the experience was over and we parted ways and made plans for the next visit.

For as long as I could remember, this was the typical family dining experience. Mostly, we ate the standard American diet and enjoyed large quantities of food at each meal. We ate this way for many years, and it never seemed like we were eating too many unhealthy foods or overeating. In fact, it was often considered an accomplishment to eat everything on the plate and finish more quickly. Although the quality of the foods we ate was often very good, there was little thought given to improving nutrition and, more importantly, portion control.

Looking back, the latter was one of the important factors that eventually led to the decline in health of some of my immediate family. For a long time, I wondered why some of my adult family members, including my dad, were overweight or borderline obese. Was it something that just happens when people get older? When I get older am I going to have a belly that hangs over my waistline? After meals, am I going to have the same trouble getting in and out of chairs? As a young man, I was often puzzled by these questions. I also wondered about my Dad. For as long as I remembered, he had a special black pouch attached just below his stomach to help him go to the bathroom. Because he had had it for many years, he was used to it and it seemed normal. I later learned that his brother also had the same special pouch and lived normally with it. As a growing teen, I wondered if something like that would happen to me someday. I did not understand why they had to wear such a thing on their bodies for life. Years later, I learned why. An operation was performed on them because most, if not all, of their large intestines were diseased and had to be removed. For the condition they both had, a colostomy was the common surgical procedure that was performed. Understanding this, I thought to myself, perhaps I should be more careful about what I eat.

During my junior year in high school, my dad was diagnosed with a form of cancer known as Non-Hodgkin's lymphoma. At the time, those were just powerful sounding words that did not mean much to me. In fact, I truly believed he was a fighter and would beat this cancer or whatever it was the doctors called it. Since my brothers were away at school and my mom was working during the day, I was asked to drive him to receive treatments at a renowned hospital in Manhattan. As I was barely driving a few months, the act of driving to the city seemed daunting. However, I thought this would help, so naturally, I volunteered.

Although he was receiving radiation treatments and seemed okay at the time, I had no idea how costly and debilitating the disease was or how painful and uncomfortable it was for him. I wondered about the nature of the treatments he received. What effect(s) were they having on his body? He was being treated in one of the best cancer facilities in the country. So why does he come home in more pain? These were difficult questions to answer because I did not understand the effects of the disease and the treatments he was receiving. As far as his diet went, I had no idea what role it played, if any, in improving his chances to overcome this painful disease. I remained optimistic and continued to take him in for the treatments. However, by the summer of 1983, my dad's condition took a turn for the worse. He was admitted to the same hospital in Manhattan, and it was decided that he receive a more intense therapeutic regimen consisting of chemotherapy and radiation. In reality, I had no idea how ill he was and continued going to school, playing drums in the school band, and playing music with my friends after school. That fall, I visited him at the hospital or called to help raise his spirits. He always expressed how much he loved me. However, late that October, his struggle with cancer ended. Sadly, my dad was gone at the age of 55.

For several years, the loss of my dad felt strange and uncomfortable, and it took awhile for me to understand how his lifestyle was related to his illness and death. Although I did not change my diet or lifestyle very much, the experience left a big impression. Until that time, I had little interest in eating more healthfully or in nutrition. It seemed important, but I was not sure how. Unintentionally, this experience led me to learn more about the relationship between foods, nutrition, and health. My journey began about 10 years later, when I discovered an interesting radio show that changed my life.

The 1990's were a very busy and interesting time in my life. In addition to gigs playing drums and singing in different bands in the evenings, I worked a day job as a computer programmer. Because I was working day and night to pay the bills, I developed insomnia and ignored the stressful consequences of it. During lunchtime I often eased the stress of the day by eating outside next to the car while listening to the radio. One day, while tuning-in, I found a radio program and heard a relaxing voice speaking about the benefits of health and nutrition. The radio show was called "Natural Living," and it featured new, specific, and somewhat controversial information about many different health-related topics. The show was very informative, and the host shared many interesting ideas and insights about living a healthy lifestyle. I listened each day to learn new and interesting information on topics that included everything from the latest scientific research on health and nutrition, foods and supplements, and recipes to the environment and natural medicines. It also featured interviews with health professionals, chefs, naturopathic doctors, farmers, scientific researchers, MDs, herbalists, and spiritual healers. There was so much new information to learn, and I began to question my own ideas about diet and lifestyle. I also read books and periodicals on natural health and about the healing properties of whole foods. However, before applying this knowledge, I faced one of the biggest challenges of my life.

During the Thanksgiving holiday of 2001, I was on a plane headed back to New York after a visit to North Carolina. As it was the first time it had happened, I remember it vividly. In addition to having chronic insomnia and being tired much of the time, I felt nervous and uncomfortable. While sitting in my seat, I felt a noticeable shortness of breath and my palms were cold and moist. As the discomfort progressed, my breath became shallower and I felt light-headed and confused. In addition, my heart pounded uncontrollably, my pulse rate increased and raced out of control. I also felt a lump in my throat and a throbbing pain in my chest and a tingling sensation running down my left arm. Was I experiencing symptoms of a heart attack? Nothing like this had happened to me before, and I was confused by the whole experience. Thankfully, after about 30 minutes, the symptoms went away and I felt much better. At first I was not sure what happened. I found out later that I had experienced a severe panic attack, and though it resembled a heart attack, was not fatal. Since it was the first time it happened, I was not very concerned and dismissed it as a simple case of nerves. I went about my life as usual and didn't think much of it. However, less than a week later, I awoke to another severe panic attack. They often occurred randomly and then passed just the same. In an effort to improve my overall health, I began learning about panic attacks and different ways to lower stress, and decided to change my diet.

Initially, my diet tended to be higher in carbohydrates from pastas, brown rice, whole grain breads, cereals, and an occasional green salad. For snacking, I ended up addicted to high-carb energy bars, granola cereals, and eating out at diners after a late night gig. Eventually, I tried adding more fresh vegetables, salads, fruits, and cut down on dairy and meats. As I understood more about panic attacks, I was better able to manage them with an improved diet and by focusing on lowering stress. There were no easy answers as to why they happened and much of the information I encountered for treating panic attacks was about managing the severity and the use of medications, and little about cures. Patience is definitely a necessary part of any healing process. However, I was not very good at being patient. In fact, I was mostly impatient when it came to taking care of my own health. In the next few years, as far as I could tell, my symptoms went back and forth between better and worse, and I felt that there was not much that could be done.

After attending a lecture by a chiropractor one day in 2002, I learned some interesting facts about how the nervous system works and how panic attacks are somehow related to nervous system imbalances. After an initial consultation, I started with regular, monthly adjustments. I thought I was onto something that would help lessen the severity and the frequency of the panic attacks or at least help me sleep better. Thankfully, the adjustments seemed to help, and I felt my sleep was improving.

Living and working in New York was difficult, and with the high cost of living there each month, I was working day and night to keep up. By the spring of 2002, I wanted a change from this stressful lifestyle and try another place to live. At that time, I had an opportunity to move to Louisville, Kentucky, and I thought it would be a good chance to lower the financial and physical work stress I was dealing with, and focus on changing my lifestyle. Overall, the smaller-sized city was more affordable, friendly, more livable, and I decided to relocate that summer.

However, despite moving, the panic attacks and increasing insomnia continued to be part of my daily life. The symptoms I experienced intensified and I did not have the financial resources to afford regular chiropractic care. My daily life in this unfamiliar new place felt like being stuck on some sort of merry-go-round and not being able to jump off. Unfortunately, the ride was not very merry.

After a few months in Louisville, I found regular work and acquired health insurance. At least this was a step in the right direction. At first, I saw different doctors who ran a battery of tests to determine the status of my health. Fortunately, the test results did not show anything life threatening, and I was diagnosed with general anxiety and chronic insomnia. Although the news was helpful, I still had a number of very uncomfortable and aggravating symptoms in my life 24/7. As part of the conventional medical doctor's diagnosis, anxiety medications, basic dietary changes, and stress reduction techniques were suggested.

Not being satisfied with the recommendations, I began researching and trying natural approaches to make progress toward improving my health. Although trying some of these things definitely helped, the lack of focus, patience, and financial resources I had at the time made it very difficult to make steady progress. In short, I was running from one health practitioner to another, and was too uncomfortable and impatient to stick with their recommendations. To make matters worse, I became obsessed with getting better and, as a result, stayed up every night studying articles on the internet about my symptoms. This made the stress and insomnia worse, and a decent nights' sleep next to impossible.

By the end of 2004, my symptoms were clearly becoming worse, and everyday life became a lot more difficult to manage. Aside from the ongoing sleep deprivation, I suffered from the following: relentless heart palpitations, ringing in the ears, fatigue and exhaustion, weakness, weight-loss, digestive and immune conditions, breathing difficulty, and was at the lowest point emotionally. To top things off, I continued having random and severe panic attacks. Some, which happened while working, were so bad I was taken by ambulance to the emergency room for further examination. Finally, after a major panic episode while performing at the Kentucky State Fair, I decided to stop playing, slow down, and focus completely on getting better. I knew I needed help and I reached out to family, friends and support groups for guidance. A few people in particular; my Mom and Great-Aunt Betty (to whom this book is dedicated), a good friend Mike Bernier, and a local chiropractor, Jeff Lagree had an important role in my recovery. Honestly, if it were not for the incredible patience, understanding, support, and love of these people, and the other health practitioners who did their best to help, I would not have made it through.

Starting out with Dr. LaGree, I had adjustments three times per week, and I tried some nutritional supplements, herbs, and foods recommended by a naturopathic doctor. Initially, it was made clear there was no guarantee that I would get better or improve very much. At first, the results of the chiropractic therapy were minimal, and I had many of the same symptoms. Fortunately, by the beginning of the fourth month, some of the major symptoms began to diminish and my sleep quality was steadily improving. Instead of one or two hours per night, the sleep duration slowly increased to four, five, and six hours. By the beginning of the sixth month of treatments, the panic attacks were not as intense and did not occur as often. In addition, the breathing difficulty was less severe and I felt my digestion was improving. With each passing month, I became stronger. In fact, in addition to walking each day, I started light jogging for short distances. Overall, the combination of things I was doing was having a positive impact on my recovery and, more importantly, I felt more optimistic about my health and my life than before.

As I felt better and stronger, I prepared more daily meals from scratch. I modified my diet to include a variety of fresh or lightly steamed vegetables, fruit smoothies, salads, and green juices in the daily routine. As I learned more about my cravings for sweets, I focused on reducing or eliminating all processed foods with added sugars or very sweet fruits. Not surprisingly, it was during this time I developed a sincere interest in food and cooking. However, one of the most influential experiences that led me down the path to becoming a chef happened purely by chance.

While working at a local health food store, some regular customers recommended I try going to different potlucks in the area. There was one in particular that was geared toward preparing dishes using more alkalizing foods and raw foods. After attending my first alkalarian potluck, I was so impressed I decided to learn more about preparing recipes using these kinds of foods. The food was tasty, simple to prepare and, more importantly, I liked the way I felt after eating it. The main difference between this type of potluck and others I attended was much more of a focus on preparing health promoting alkaline dishes and sharing ideas and information about nutrition and the how people felt about this kind of lifestyle. During these potlucks there were also brief presentations by some of the participants about the positive changes they had experienced. There was also an enthusiasm and excitement in the people that was unlike any I had encountered at other potlucks. After attending a few of them, I began eating this way and started creating new recipes using alkaline foods. Many of the recipes in this book are end results of those experiences.

In the summer of 2006, I volunteered a few days a week in the kitchen at the local Salvation Army. After learning of a culinary training class given there, I enrolled that fall. The class was excellent, and it offered an opportunity to learn basic culinary concepts, skills and practice cooking alongside some great local chefs. In addition to helping out in the kitchen at the shelter, the culinary program offered an internship with a local restaurant after graduation. Since I already had an interest in health and nutrition, taking the class helped me discover a passion for healthy cooking, and which direction to take my cooking skills. By the end of 2006, I was nearly symptom-free and, after graduating from the culinary class, was ready to work in a restaurant. It was an exciting time, and I felt a true sense of hope and renewal in my life.

In addition to the chiropractic therapy and the other natural therapies I tried while recovering, there were a few major discoveries that contributed to the direction I took in developing recipes and eating in general. One was more scientific, the other was culinary, and each was introduced by two good friends. The scientific discovery was about the concept of pH or acid-alkaline balance and the role that it plays in the state of health in the body. The relationship between pH-balance and health has been well documented in the scientific literature for well over 100 years. Based upon some readings from traditional Chinese and Ayurveda medicine texts, research of Professor Antoine Bechamp, Dr. Bernard Jensen, Dr. Max Gerson, Dr. Robert O. Young and others, I discovered that the blood and tissues of the human body require a slightly alkaline pH (between 7.2 – 7.4) to be healthy and balanced. More specifically, the foods we eat and the substances that they break down into in the body have a direct effect on its pH-balance. Based upon research proposed by the above researchers, most, if not all, foods made from animal sources and processed foods cause a more acidic environment in the body. This occurs because excess metabolic acids are produced by the body when it digests these types of foods. Regular consumption or over-consumption of these acid-forming foods in the diet can (over time) cause imbalances which weaken the body's immune system. More importantly, the weakening of the body's defenses is further magnified by chronic stress, lack of exercise and proper detoxification, emotional stress, etc., and this combination can lead to chronic illness, disease, or pre-mature aging.

Putting some of these ideas together, I had a better understanding of some of the underlying causes for my illness. In response to the dilemma I faced, it became clear that I had nothing to lose by applying some of the knowledge of pH-balance to my diet, lifestyle, and to developing new recipes.

While learning about acid-alkaline balance, I discovered an interesting educational tool called microscopy. This involves the examination, by a trained professional microscopist, of the blood in live and dried form using a phase contrast and bright field microscope. By being able to look at the physical condition of my blood, I learned valuable information about the quality of my health which helped me focus on ways to improve it. As a result, I had a better understanding of the foundation of my health and how it is related to diet and lifestyle changes. By applying concepts of pH-balancing, drinking more pure, filtered, alkaline pH-water, and eating more alkaline rich vegetables and fruits, nuts, and seeds, etc., I found a simpler way to take better care of myself, and it was not too difficult or expensive. Plant-based foods such as chlorophyll-rich vegetables and low sugar fruits are well-documented to help alkalize and maintain a healthy pH level of the blood and tissues of the body. By incorporating a higher percentage of these foods over several months and monitoring my pH level using pH hydrion strips, the results were quite significant. Months later, when I had another microscopy examination, I compared results with the first one. The changes in the quality and health of my blood were undeniable and, most importantly, I had more energy, felt much better, and had a healthier outlook on life. In all, my food intake and lifestyle changed for the better, and I had the physical results and renewed energy to show for it.

In the kitchen, I began working on recipes that contained more alkalizing foods and learned more about food cravings; namely how sweet cravings affected my behavior. With the help of regular seasonal juice feasts (juice fasting), I dramatically lowered my sweet cravings. I also learned how to incorporate a few dashes of unprocessed natural sea salt, different spice combinations, and a squeeze of lemon, lime, or adding a sea vegetable to enhance the flavor of recipes. As a result, my sense of taste felt more accurate and balanced. Naturally sweet vegetables and low sugar fruits had a richer flavor and were sweet enough to be satisfying to my taste. This turned out to be a significant breakthrough. Ultimately, the dietary changes I made after the juice fasts helped adjust my sense of taste to enjoy the true flavor(s) of real, unprocessed foods. By having a better sense of taste, I became more aware of how to put foods together to create new recipes.

When I started creating recipes, a friend had introduced me to quinoa. I had never heard of it and it quickly became an important ingredient in guiding me to create a new recipe. I loved it immediately and it sparked a new curiosity and passion for cooking. In fact, "Magic Quinoa" was the very first recipe I created and it is included in this book. For this reason, quinoa has always had a special significance. Since creating "Magic Quinoa", I have made it countless times for friends, family, and for cooking classes and potlucks. Many have remarked how quinoa's light, nutty taste and fluffy texture are very satisfying. Ultimately, creating this recipe allowed me to experiment with spices, create new flavors and textures, and it was my first success in the kitchen as an up-and-coming chef.

Today, I am symptom-free, have not had a panic attack in over five years, and really enjoy my work as a chef creating and demonstrating recipes, educating others about healthy cuisine, and sharing information about food and nutrition. I enjoy spending time in the kitchen tinkering with different foods, developing new recipes, and researching the vast scientific information on the benefits of different foods. In addition, I can often be found jogging to and from the store for produce, completing a local marathon, or playing drums, and performing with some fantastic musicians. In fact, I feel younger, more energetic, and happier than I have in years, and I have learned to take better care of myself. The quality of my health, energy and vitality lost during those difficult times has returned in leaps and bounds, and I am completely grateful for where I am today.

As a result of overcoming a health challenge, I learned much about the healing properties of living foods. Of course it's not necessary that someone have an illness to benefit from these recipes. Anyone seeking better meal options can try them. I hope by reading this story you have a deeper appreciation of the experience of living through an illness, or through the illness of a loved one. I hope you find some of that experience, along with the following recipes and informational resources, a source of inspiration to help guide you toward improving the quality of your life.

In closing, I would like to leave you with a few random thoughts that will inspire you in your journey to a happier, healthier, and more prosperous life:

Give yourself a gift every day; the gift of good nutrition.

Take your time, chew your food well, and enjoy it.

The greatest wealth is the quality of your health.

Doctors do not make *you* better. They entertain *you* while *you* do the healing.

Being a patient, patient is usually much better.

By building healthy cells you build healthy tissues, organs, bones, etc.

Nothing tastes as good as good health feels.

It's okay to go hungry from time to time; especially while walking through airports or malls.

Under-spice the recipe; you can always add more.

Get at least 15 minutes of sun on your face daily. Dawn and dusk are especially good times for it. Of course, it's much better to avoid looking directly at it.

Green foods aren't so bad. Your taste buds just don't know it yet.

Drink your food and chew your drinks.

It's hard to be sick; a lot harder than being well.

Living foods provide living energy to a living body.

Serve each meal with at least 51% raw foods or more on the plate.

Play some of the music of Mozart, Chopin, or Gershwin, while cooking or eating.

Laughter lifts your mood, heals the soul, and aids digestion. Have a good laugh each day.

Give and receive the most important vitamin each day; vitamin-**L**ove

Drink half your weight (in ounces) of pure, filtered or natural spring (directly from the source water throughout each day.

Attend a local, plant-based potluck this weekend.

Leave your car home on a nice day and walk or bike to the market instead.

Adopting a better food lifestyle takes practice. Practice better food choices each day.

Buy local, seasonal produce or eat at restaurants that specialize in it.

Don't forget to add in some **t**ender, **l**oving, **c**are, spice to every recipe.

Sleep deeply and dream well every night.

Breathe deeply, in and out.

Hang in there!

Part II
Getting Started

Utensil Checklist:

- Chef's knife – 8" blade, hi-carbon steel with sharpener
- Paring knife – 2" or 3" blade
- Serrated knife – short and long
- Cutting boards – small and large, non-porous polypropylene or bamboo
- Measuring cups – (sizes) ¼ cup through 2 cup
- Measuring spoons – (sizes) 1/8 tsp. through 1 Tbsp.
- Flat Spatula – silicon and/or wooden
- Skillet – 8", 10" or 12" Stainless steel, ceramic, or corning ware
- Wok – 12" or 14" for the stove top or stainless portable electric
- Saucepans – 1 quart, 5 quart stainless steel or corning ware (check eBay)
- Baking sheet – non-stick, small and large
- Colander – stainless steel or wire mesh
- Cheese cloth
- Peeler
- Whisk – small and large
- Box grater
- Can opener
- Apple corer-divider
- Large wooden spoon and slotted spoon
- Set of mixing bowls – small, medium, and large
- Set of small and large prep bowls
- Storage containers and bags
- Steamer
- Glass mason jars for soup stock – pint or quart sized jars

- Variable speed blender – 450 watts or higher or a Vita-mix

- Coffee grinder for grinding herbs, seeds or grains

- Juicer – centrifugal type (Juiceman, Jack Lalanne, Breville, etc.) or masticating type (Omega, Champion, Green Star, etc.)

- Food dehydrator – Nesco, Ronco, Weston, Excalibur, etc.

<u>Spices Checklist: (organic where available)</u>

- Sea salt – Redmond's, pink Himalayan, Celtic
- Black or white pepper – from freshly ground peppercorns
- Basil leaves*
- Bay Leaf
- Chili powder
- Chives*
- Cinnamon (fresh ground)
- Coriander seeds or powder
- Cumin seeds or powder
- Curry powder – Masala, Madras, Muchi, etc.
- Dill weed*
- Fennel seeds* or powder
- Garlic powder*
- Ginger root powder*
- Herbs De Provence
- Italian seasoning
- Nutmeg (freshly ground kernel)
- Onion powder
- Oregano leaves*
- Paprika
- Pumpkin pie spice
- Rosemary leaves* or powder
- Sage leaves*
- Tarragon leaves*
- Thyme leaves*
- Turmeric root powder*
- Vanilla beans* or extract

* = Use the fresh variety whenever possible

*Fats and Oils Checklist: (Organic, Unrefined and Cold-Pressed
Varieties)
Non-cooking oils:
- Argan oil (P)
- Black Currant seed oil (P)
- Borage oil (P)
- Extra virgin coconut oil (S)
- Extra virgin olive oil (M)
- Evening primrose oil (P)
- Fish oils (P)
- Flaxseed oil (P)
- Grapeseed oil (P)
- Hempseed oil (M)
- Pumpkin seed oil (M)
- Sacha Inchi oil (P).

Cooking oils:
- Almond oil (M)
- Avocado oil (M)
- Extra virgin coconut oil (S)
- Grapeseed oil
- Light, virgin, or extra virgin olive oil (M)
- Peanut oil (P)
- Rice bran oil (M)
- Sesame oil (P)
- Sunflower oil (P)
- Walnut oil (M).

Key: (M) = Monounsaturated, (P) = Polyunsaturated, (S) = Saturated

Note: Some oils can be used in both non-cooking and cooking applications. An important thing to remember is the following oils: almond (420°F), avocado (500°F), coconut (350°F), grapeseed (390°F), rice bran oil (490°F), sesame (410°F), walnut (400°F), etc., can handle up to their listed cooking temperatures before reaching their smoke point, breaking down, and turning rancid (spoiling).

*In general, it's best to use fats and oils in moderation and avoid over heating. Please use them as needed or substitute with vegetable stock in daily cooking.

Tips on how to use this book

I. Making vegetable stock

As you read through the recipes in this book, you'll notice the word stock bowl is frequently listed in the utensils section. By collecting and saving your vegetable clippings in the stock bowl and making your own vegetable stock, you will benefit in the following ways:

- It's a simple-to-do, no cost way to make homemade vegetable stock.
- The stock contains more beneficial nutrition from a variety of vegetables.
- For those interested in lowering calories in recipes or who are following food lifestyle programs like *The Engine 2 Diet* or *Forks Over Knives*, it's a terrific substitute for cooking oils. Feel free to use it in place of olive oil or sesame oil, etc., or wherever you desire. In general for most recipes, use about ¼ cup of stock or more to substitute for the oil. As it absorbs and evaporates more quickly than cooking oil, you may need to add more stock to finish cooking a particular recipe.
- You can use it to enhance the flavor of many of your recipes and to create a new flavor base for soups, sauces, marinates or to create new recipes.
- By composting the leftover vegetable clippings, you do a little extra to help the environment and your garden too.
- It lasts a long time and can be stored in a properly sealed mason jar for about 2 to 3 weeks in the fridge or longer in the freezer. For long term freezing, be sure to use a heavy-duty plastic container or jars more suitable for long term freezing.

II. Minimal cooking and vegetables

Here are some suggestions on preparing and cooking the recipes. If you are already a well-seasoned cook and understand basic nutrition, that's wonderful and you can go ahead and dig into the recipes. However, if not, here are a few basic tips to keep in mind.

- Remembering that the nutrition in foods is lost due to heat from the cooking process, it's important to be aware of the color, texture, flavor and aroma while cooking. A good indication of the temperature of the food is revealed by how warm it is to the touch.
  If the temperature is too high, you will not be able to handle it. With that in mind, taste the recipes occasionally and keep the heat from getting too high for too long.
- With a few exceptions, raw or lightly steamed vegetables offer a richer flavor, color, crisp texture, and better nutrition. To minimize the loss of these important elements during cooking, use lower stove and baking temperatures, and light steaming where possible.

- In general, sprouted vegetables, whole grains, and legumes provide more nutrition density per calorie and ease of digestion than their cooked forms. However, their cooked forms do offer important nutrients, fiber, and are good to include in recipes to help keep you going in colder climates.

III. Raw versus cooked

There is an ongoing debate about raw versus cooked foods, and there are many great recipe books using raw foods or cooked foods exclusively. There's no doubt that eating more raw foods daily, at least 51% or higher at each meal, has many benefits to support a healthy body. This book contains a combination of both. To clarify, raw foods are foods that are not heated to an internal temperature over 115° F. Most of the breakdown of vital enzymes, phytochemicals, proteins, and other nutrients occur at or beyond this temperature. With that in mind, here are a few simple suggestions to help your daily food lifestyle and get the best of both worlds:

- To help reach your daily raw food goal, prepare either the "Green Machine" or the "AM Attitude Protein Smoothie," or both, every day. It's the simplest way to get plenty of fresh raw fruits and vegetables, and takes only minutes to prepare.
- If you add a simple green salad, the "Mango Chunky Salsa," "Whole-You-Guacamole," "Banana Nut Torte," or "Not Your Average Cucumber Salad," etc., you've already reached the raw food goal for the day.
- To round out the day's menu, pick any of the cooked recipes like, "Luscious Lentil Soup" with "Baked Sweets" and include a small mixed green salad for lunch or dinner.
- For snacks, there are many delicious and satisfying raw food bars with no added sugars, unhealthy or refined oils, artificial flavors, colors, and preservatives, etc. I have listed several websites these on the web resources page and the snacks "On the Go Quick and Simple Snack Ideas" recipe page. Feel free to look them up. These really help you save time, come in handy to have on a busy day, are great for travel outings, and make practical sense to add to the kids' school lunch.

IV. Juicing

One of the easiest ways to increase your daily intake of raw foods and alkalizing foods is by juicing fresh organic or local, vegetables, fruits, or wheat grass. Ultimately, the nutrition from fresh juices requires little digestive effort, fills the body with enzymes, vitamins, minerals, antioxidants, phytochemicals, and helps the body cleanse and detoxify on a deeper level.

I highly recommend trying fresh green juices at a local juice bar or juicing at home. By doing so, you'll enjoy the many vital benefits nature offers the body; both inside and out.

V. Sprouting
Sprouts have numerous benefits to promote health. They are some of the most alkaline forming and energizing foods available. They contain easily digestible sources of proteins, vitamins, minerals enzymes, and antioxidants, and keep the body youthful and strong. The best part is you can grow them easily at home with the following directions for 'Sprouted Out Loud Legume Salad'.

- Set aside three sprouting jars or mason jars with a cheese cloth covering the top.
- Measure out ¼ cup each of the mung beans, lentils, garbanzos, and fill each jar.
- Fill each jar with at least two or more cups of filtered water and a dash of sea salt.
- Cover each jar with a kitchen towel and store on top of the refrigerator or counter overnight.
- The next day, drain the water, rinse the beans in a colander a few times, and drain well. This should be done at least two times per day or the sprouts may spoil or develop mold.
- Cover the jars with a towel, repeat the above step for the next two days or until you see the tails form. Typically, they are finished when the tail is ¼" or longer.
- When finished, make sure to keep them dry, refrigerated, and in a sealed container. They will keep well for up to five days.

VI. Eating more alkaline forming foods
Since this may be a new area for many people, I have included a chart of both acid and alkaline forming foods. Although the chart is not all-inclusive, it will help you get started. Feel free to make a copy of it, put it on your iPhone or computer, and use it while shopping at the market or when ordering at a restaurant. Try including at least one or more of the foods from the alkaline forming list daily. Since this book contains many recipes with these foods, you have options to try each day. This will assist you in making better daily food choices so you can get the most out of eating health-promoting foods in the long run. Ultimately, every day you are making your health a priority and that makes a positive difference in your life.

VII. Healthy eating can be fun.
Sometimes all of the talk about what foods to eat and all the nutrition information out there can be confusing, controversial, or even distressing. Yes, it's important to

understand that getting proper nutrition every day is important and peoples' individual needs are different.

It's also important to know that foods have a big effect on energy, mood, and how you feel. The scientific information and research available on nutrition can be helpful to you in your journey to better health. However, that does not mean discovering better eating habits won't be delicious and fun. If this book introduces at least one new food or recipe that you absolutely enjoy, that creates a wonderful new experience in your life. That's the fun about food.

VIII. Transitioning: One step at a time.
One of the important things to clarify for those beginning to transition their dietary habits is to start with small steps. Prepare one home-made meal each day or every other day and include fresh, local or organic produce, and natural ingredients. For those with very busy lifestyles and less time to shop and prepare, try a local health food store's prepared foods section or organic salad bar. These can help jump-start your healthy eating habits.

Starting out, it can be quite overwhelming to make drastic changes regarding your food choices. As a result, you may lose interest because you either end up trying too hard and give up or realize it's not fun or practical enough to make too many changes in a short period of time. That's why it's very important to start small and practice making better choices each day. The body has a tremendous capacity to heal itself and, by making your health a priority, improving the nutrition it receives will have a cumulative and positive impact in the long run. So, please take one step at a time and build on your progress.

IX. Water you talking about?
We are all born with beautifully soft and supple skin (about 90% water). The health of our body organs, tissues, and fluids rely on clean water. It's no small miracle that water is the primary drink to maintain the foundation of optimal health. As a general rule, build up to drinking half your weight in ounces of clean, filtered, local spring, or more alkaline pH water (7.5 – 9.5) throughout each day.

Another thing:
The occasional "oops I shouldn't have eaten that" is realistic and happens to all of us from time to time. If you are in reasonably good health, it's perfectly fine and sensible to try something new, a favorite comfort food, or enjoy a really decadent dessert now and then. These experiences can be really fun, enjoyable and even inspirational. It's important to know that it's okay to enjoy these things on occasion. The main idea to keep in mind is the 80/20 rule. By choosing and or preparing at least 80% of your daily meals containing raw or lightly cooked

unprocessed, non-GMO, additive-free, local, or organically produced foods, and 20% or less of processed packaged foods, canned foods, overcooked foods, there's a much greater potential to make steady, realistic progress toward improving the foundation of your health. Eventually, by eating better, your body will tell you what works and what doesn't. You will become more confident choosing or preparing delicious and healthy foods that taste good to you and make you feel good. This is how you can improve the way you feel and hence make steady progress to a better quality lifestyle. Remember, nothing tastes as good as good health feels.

A note about preparation times:
Please note that the total prep times are estimated and some of the more seasoned home cooks or experienced chefs may finish sooner than those who are just beginners. Understanding that no two cooks do things the same way, I did my best to come up with an average time to complete the recipes, and enlisted friends and family members to test many of them out. Basically, the time for each recipe is measured from the time all the ingredients are in place to the time it is placed on the platter or serving dish. Of course, the more you get used to doing your favorite recipes, I'm sure the overall time(s) will decrease.

Part III
The Recipes

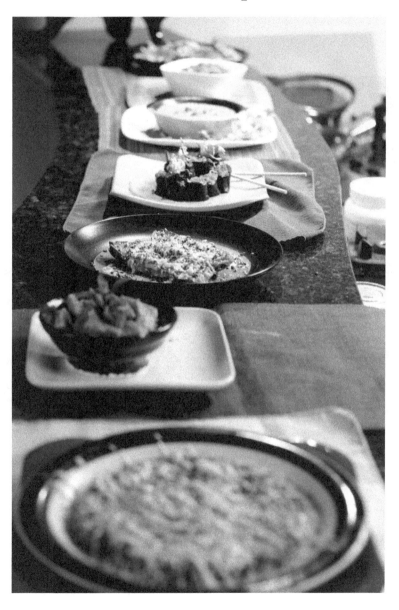

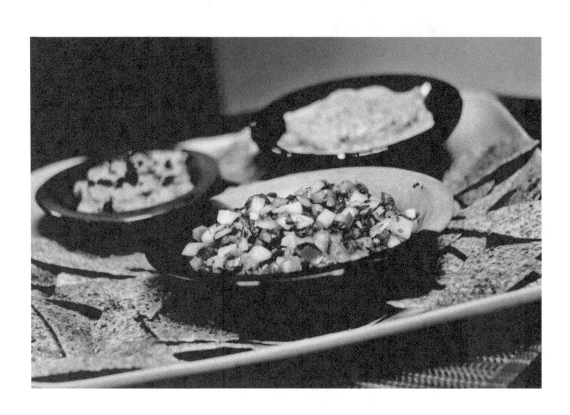

Appealing Appetizers

Bang Zoom Manna

Chunky Mango Salsa

Not Your Average Cucumber Salad

Sprouted Out Loud Legume Salad

Sun-dried Tomato Hummus

Sunny Pressed Salad

Whole–You–Guacamole

Bang Zoom Manna

Named after an ancient food of the Essenes, manna bread uses soaked and sprouted whole grains to help improve their digestibility. This tasty appetizer offers a simple and enjoyable way to get a daily amount of brain supporting omega -3 and monounsaturated fats. It's also a good source of protein, minerals like calcium, magnesium, and iodine, and fiber. It makes a great snack, appetizer, and can be served with a green salad, soup, or your favorite dip. Prep time: 15 to 20 minutes.

Ingredients: Organic or local
Manna bread – 1 loaf, any variety (freezer section of natural grocery section)
Wakame flakes (sea vegetable) – 1 tsp., soaked & expanded (international food section)
Flaxseed oil – 1 tsp. per slice (Barlean's or Udo's Perfect oil blend)
Ground flaxseed – ½ tsp. per slice
Sea salt – lightly sprinkled over top
Avocado – 1 ripe (soft enough to spread easily)

Optional:
Extra virgin coconut oil – 1 tsp. per slice, instead of flaxseed oil
Cayenne powder – 1 pinch per slice
Your favorite spice or combination sprinkled over top

Utensils: Serrated knife, cutting board, bowl for soaking wakame, measuring spoons, toaster oven or oven w/baking sheet, pastry brush or spoon, spreading knife, wire mesh strainer.

Directions:
- Pre-thaw the manna before slicing.
- Soak 1 tsp. wakame flakes in a bowl of water and allow a few minutes to expand.
- Pre-heat oven or toaster oven to 300.
- Using a serrated knife, cut the manna loaf into several ½" wide slices.
- Arrange them in one layer on a baking sheet and toast until light brown and slightly crispy (about 10 minutes). Remove and let cool for a few minutes.
- Using a wire mesh strainer, thoroughly drain the expanded wakame over the sink.
- Place the toasted manna on a cutting board, spread on the flaxseed oil, sea salt, spices, a light spread of ripe avocado, top with a piece or two of the sea weed, a few dashes of ground flaxseed, and your favorite spice.

- Cut the pieces into halves or quarters, plate, and serve as appetizers or party hors d'oeuvres.

Chunky Mango Salsa

In a short time, you can prepare a healthfully versatile snack recipe for many occasions. If you are looking for a dish that satisfies snack cravings, will not affect your waistline, is affordable and easy-to-prepare, mango salsa is one of the best foods to have around. It's chock full of lycopene, beta carotene, vitamin C and bioflavinoids, iron, antioxidants, and many more immune system supporting nutrients. Prep time: 25 to 30 minutes.
Makes about 1 quart.

Ingredients: Organic, local or seasonal
Vine ripe tomatoes – 4 to 5 large, cored, seeded and small diced
Sweet or Vidalia onion – 1 medium sized, small diced
Green pepper - 1 medium sized, cored, seeded, and small diced
Jalapeño* – 1, cored, seeded & minced
Serrano* pepper – 1, cored, seeded, and minced
Mango – 1, fresh, ripe, peeled, pitted, and small diced
Garlic cloves - 3 cloves, minced
Cilantro - ½ bunch, rough chopped small
Lime – 1, freshly juiced
Apple cider vinegar - 2 Tbsps., organic, raw variety
Sea salt – 1 tsp.
Cumin – 1 tsp.

Optional:
Habanero* pepper – 1, small, minced
Cayenne powder - 1 to 2 pinches

Utensils: Chef's knife, paring knife or small serrated knife, cutting board, food processor**, large mixing bowl, mixing spoon, measuring spoons, peeler, mango pitter, compost bin, a pair of food service gloves, stock bowl.

Directions:
- Rinse and drain the produce in the sink.
- Cut the vegetables in order as above and place them in a large mixing bowl.
- Add in the lime juice, cider vinegar, sea salt, cumin, and mix well.
- Taste and adjust seasonings if desired.
- Serve chilled with lots of 'Crunchies'.
- Keep refrigerated in a sealed container until ready to use. Stores well for 7 to 8 days.

*Caution: If you are sensitive to handling hot peppers, be sure to use a pair of food service gloves. Also, avoid touching your eyes, face, or other extremities while handling. After handling them, remove gloves, wash hands, and dry them well with a towel.

****Tip**: If you prefer the convenience of a food processor, rough chop the vegetables, add them to the food processor, and pulse the ingredients a few times or until desired size is reached.

An important thing to note here is to keep an eye on how chunky or smooth you want the finished salsa.

Add Your Own Recipe Ideas Here:

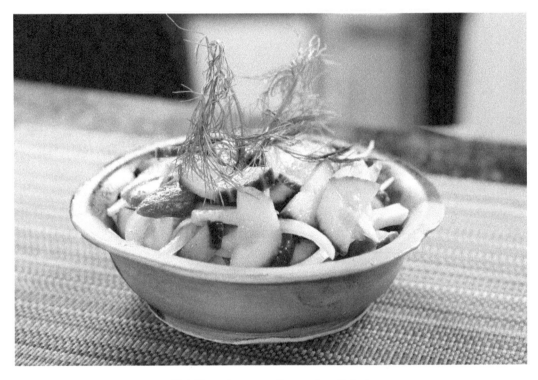

Not Your Average Cucumber Salad

Not Your Average Cucumber Salad

From the last minute dinner gathering to an impromptu salad for snacking, this appetizing, easy–to-prepare recipe can be table ready in less than 15 minutes. Each time I prepare this dish for an event I'm amazed to see both adults and kids enjoying a dish containing raw onions. In addition its enjoyable flavor, this recipe supplies significant amounts of beneficial nutrients like: potassium, lycopene, silica, water, vitamin A, vitamin C, folate, fiber, and phytonutrients. Prep time: 15 minutes. Serves 2 to 4.

Ingredients: Organic, local or seasonal
English cucumber (or regular) – 1 lg. or 2 med. sized, sliced into ¼" half moons
Beefsteak or plum tomatoes – 2, cored, sliced into thin wedges
Sweet onion – ½, cored, julienne (very thin, stick-like slices)
Fennel bulb – ½ a bulb, julienne (very thin, stick-like slices)
Raw apple cider vinegar – 2 to 3 Tbsps.
Sea salt – 2 tsp.
Cumin – 1 tsp.
White pepper – 1/8 tsp.

Optional:
Cayenne powder – 1 dash
Red or yellow pepper – ½ cup, medium diced

Utensils: Chef's knife, cutting board, measuring cup and spoons, colander, large mixing bowl, mixing spoon, and stock bowl.

Directions:
- Rinse and drain all the vegetables, and prepare them as above.
- Using a tablespoon, scoop and remove the cucumber seeds if desired.
- Place the prepared vegetables into a large mixing bowl, pour in the cider vinegar, all seasonings, and mix well.
- Taste and adjust seasonings if desired.
- Plate and serve chilled.
- Refrigerate in a sealed container and finish within 4 to 5 days.

Sprouted Out Loud Legume Salad

Sprouting unlocks the nutritional arsenal contained within foods, helps improve digestion, and absorption. If you are looking for some of the most nutritionally dense and energizing foods on the planet, look no further than sprouted seeds, beans, and legumes. In nature, sprouted foods offer a huge nutrient potential and this recipe highlights their flavors and textures. This nutritionally rich dish offers an abundance of enzymes, complete protein, vitamins, minerals, antioxidants, and phytonutrients. Prep time: 10 to 15 minutes.

Ingredients: Organic, local or seasonal

Sprouted mung beans – ½ cup (pre-sprouted pkg. from produce area)
Sprouted green lentils – ½ cup (pre-sprouted pkg. from produce area)
Sprouted garbanzo beans – ½ cup (pre-sprouted pkg. from produce area)
Green onions – ¼ cup, rough chopped
Shredded carrots – ½ cup
Tamari (wheat–free variety) – 2 tsp.
Lemon juice – ½, fresh squeezed
Extra virgin olive oil or flaxseed oil – 1 Tbsp.

Optional:

Fennel bulb – ½ bulb, rough chopped
Cayenne powder – 1 dash

Utensils: Chef's knife, cutting board, measuring cup and spoons, colander, large mixing bowl, mixing spoon, and stock bowl.

Directions:

- Sprout* (see page 21) all beans as directed below or rinse and drain the pre-packaged sprouts in a colander. After draining, pat them dry with a paper towel.
- Prepare vegetables as above and mix them with the sprouts in a large mixing bowl.
- Mix in the tamari, lemon juice, and oil.
- Taste, adjust flavor and finish with a dash or two of cayenne powder.
- Refrigerate and serve chilled.
- Makes a great addition to a mixed green salad, sandwich or wrap.
- Store in refrigerator and finish within three to five days.

Sun-dried Tomato Hummus

Hummus may be one of the most versatile foods to make for many occasions. It's easy to prepare and, if you like the rich flavor of sun-dried tomatoes, you'll enjoy making it often. Hummus, the Arabic word for chickpea, is one of the oldest food dishes in recorded history. It goes back over 7000 years. In addition to delicious flavor, this hummus recipe supplies an excellent source of protein, monounsaturated fats, fiber, vitamin C, folate, potassium, and magnesium. Prep time: 15 to 20 minutes. Makes about 3½ cups.

Ingredients: Organic, local or seasonal
Garbanzo beans (chick peas) – 1½, 15 oz. cans (or 2 full cans for a thicker finish)
Tahini – sesame seed paste (found near the nut butters) – ¼ cup
Sun-dried tomatoes - ½ cup (whole size, dry-packed variety), pre-soaked
Fresh lemon juice – ¼ cup (2 to 3 medium sized lemons)
Garlic cloves – 2, minced
Sea salt – 1 tsp.
Cumin – 1 tsp.
Extra virgin olive oil – 3 Tbsps.

Optional:
Vegetable broth or water – ¼ cup, to thin out (if desired)
Parsley – rough chopped, sprinkled for garnish
Roasted garlic cloves* – 6, roasted in the skillet with olive oil or vegetable broth
Cayenne powder – 1 or 2 pinches

Utensils: Food processor or blender, flat spatula, prep bowls, soaking bowl for sun-dried tomatoes, colander, measuring cup and spoons, cutting board, chef's knife, citrus reamer or juicer, and serving platter.

Directions:
Soak the sun-dried tomatoes in warm water until soft then drain.

Tip: To save prep time and improve the consistency of the finished hummus, use a small food processor or chopping utensil and mince the pre-soaked sun-dried tomatoes, and garlic cloves together.

- Rinse and drain the garbanzo beans in the colander.
- Add them to the food processor along with tahini, the chopped sun-dried tomatoes, garlic, lemon juice, and all seasonings.
- Pulse the food processor and gradually add in the olive oil to improve the texture.

- To ensure even mixing, occasionally scrape the sides of the food processor cup with a sturdy spatula.
- Mix until very smooth.
- Taste and adjust seasonings. If desired, add an additional Tbsp. of tahini or olive oil to improve the finished texture. If the texture is still too thick, add in a few tablespoons of stock or water.
- Remove the contents with a spatula and refrigerate in a sealed container. Stores well for up to two weeks.
- Plate and serve chilled with veggie sticks and "Crunchies".

*Variation: For a smoother texture and deeper flavor, substitute the roasted garlic cloves for the raw garlic. To roast the garlic, add 4 to 5 Tbsps. olive oil to a skillet on medium heat, add in the cloves, and stir occasionally until soft and golden brown (about 15 to 20 minutes).

Add Your Own Recipe Ideas Here:

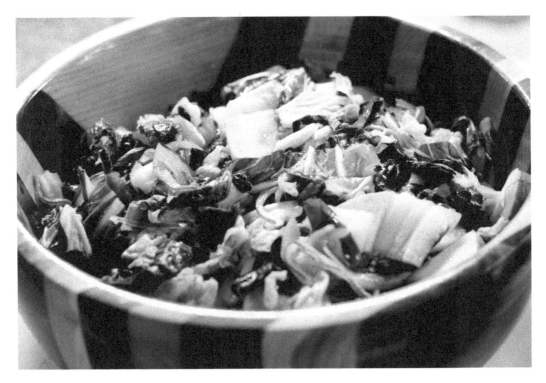

Sunny Pressed Salad

Sunny Pressed Salad

A crunchy, raw green feast of flavor! Cabbages contain sulfur containing compounds like indole-3-carbinol (I3C) and sulforaphane, etc. These substances help fight oxidative stress and inflammation, promote a healthy digestive tract, and help detoxify the body. Aside from the great nutrition, my favorite things about this salad are the flavor and the crunch. An important thing to note about this recipe is about adding the plum vinegar. It has a strong flavor so it's better to under-use it so you can always add more at the end if necessary. Prep time 20 to 25 minutes. Serves 6 to 8.

Ingredients: Organic, local or seasonal
Bok Choy - 1 head, cleaned and rinsed
Napa cabbage or savoy – 1 small head, cleaned, rinsed and cored
Red onion – 1, cored, julienne (thin, stick-like slices)
Wakame (seaweed) - 2 to 3 Tbsps., soaked and expanded
Green apples - 1 large, cored, sliced into thin wedges
Cranberries – 1 cup, dried (apple juice flavored if available)
Umeboshi plum vinegar (by Eden foods) - 4 to 5 Tbsps.

Optional:
Sprouts – mung beans, lentils or adzuki beans, mixed, etc. – 1 cup
Chopped walnuts – ½ cup

Utensils: Chef's knife, cutting board, colander, prep bowls, very large serving bowl, serving tongs, apple corer/divider, measuring cup, stock bowl, a large plate to fit over salad and a heavy book or pot to place on top of it, and some hungry people with a healthy appetite.

Directions:
- Fill the sink with water.
- Wash any debris off the cabbages, rinse the apples, and allow all to drain in a large colander.
- Set aside a bowl of water and soak the wakame until it expands. (About 5 minutes).
- Remove the stem part of each cabbage and set it aside for the stock bowl or compost.
- Rough chop the cabbage into thin, 2" to 3" long, bite size pieces, and toss them into a large serving bowl.
- Cut the onion in half, remove the skin, core, and slice into ¼" wide, thin strips, and place in serving bowl.

- Using the apple corer, slice the apple into wedges. Carefully slice each apple wedge twice (long ways) to make three equal pieces then cut them in half going across.
- Mix in the sliced apple wedges, cranberries, optional sprouts, and plum vinegar with the cabbages.
- Drain the wakame well and mix it in to finish the salad.

Finishing:
- Place a large plate (face down) on top and add a heavy pot or book on top of it to help press down on the salad.
- Place the salad into the refrigerator and allow it to chill for about 10 to 15 minutes.
- Serve chilled with a pair of wooden spoons or tongs for a nice presentation.

Tip: Save the leftover soaking water from the wakame to water the plants around the house. It's full of beneficial nutrients to help them grow.

Whole–You–Guacamole

This recipe is for the avocado lover in you. It's the classic party dish, topping or movie snack that's full of great texture, flavor, and promotes alkalinity in the body. Avocados provide an excellent source of potassium, vitamin K, fiber, and monounsaturated fats. Eating guacamole regularly offers you a timely, simple, cost effective way to enjoy a versatile dip, and maintain youthful, beautiful skin. That's the true meaning of stealth health. Prep time: 20 to 25 minutes. Makes one pint.

Ingredients: Organic, local or seasonal
Sweet or red onion – ½, small diced
Garlic cloves – 2 to 3, minced
Jalapeño pepper* – 1, cored, seeded, minced
Serrano pepper* – 1, cored, seeded, minced
Cilantro leaves (fresh) – ¼ cup, de-stemmed and rough chopped
Limes – 2, fresh juiced
Avocado – 3, ripe (soft but not squishy), and pitted
Sea salt – 1 tsp.
Cumin powder – 1 tsp.

Optional:
Tomato – 1 small, ripe plum tomato or roma – seeded and small diced
Habanera pepper* – 1, cored, seeded, minced, (for some extra heat)
Cayenne powder – a pinch or two

Utensils: Chef's knife, paring knife, cutting board, large mixing bowl, prep bowl, flat spatula, potato masher or large fork, serving bowl, citrus juicer, large spoon for scooping avocado, a pair of food service gloves, and stock bowl.

Directions:
- Cut vegetables in order as above, place in prep bowl, and juice the limes.
- Using a chef's knife, slice into the avocado horizontally (long ways) until you hit the pit. Using the palm of your hand, turn the avocado slowly in a circle and allow the knife slice around it. Go around it once until you can twist off the top to separate it into two pieces.
- Remove the inside pit by gently chopping into it and turning to remove it.
- Over a mixing bowl, scoop out avocado contents with a sturdy spoon and discard or compost the skins.

Mixing:

- Using a potato masher or large fork, lightly mash the avocado until mostly smooth.
- With a flat spatula, fold in all the prepared vegetables, any optional ingredients, seasonings, and lime juice. Taste and adjust seasonings.
- Place in a serving bowl, garnish with some chopped cilantro, and serve with veggie sticks and some "Crunchies".

Tip: If the finished texture is not thick enough, try adding in another avocado to make it '*thickerer*'. To thin out, add in an extra tsp. lime juice. Taste and adjust seasonings if desired.

Freshness tips: To help maintain freshness, place an avocado pit in with the guacamole. Cover it with clear plastic wrap, allow the plastic wrap to set on the surface of the guacamole, secure the lid, and store. This helps maintain color and freshness longer. Refrigerate and eat within 3 days.

*Caution: If your skin is sensitive to working with hot peppers, be sure to you use a pair of food service gloves while handling and preparing them. Also, be careful not to touch your eyes, exposed wounds or sensitive areas, and wash and dry hands well after working with them.

Anytime Breakfasts and Snacks

Crunchies

Crunchy Roasted Bonzo's

Get In the Groove Grapefruit Breakfast

Michael's Yummy Groats

On the Go Quick and Simple Snack Ideas

Sweet Crunchies Cereal

Toasted A.B. & J. Sandwich

Crunchies

If you crave the crunch, here's a way for you to create the perfect crunchy snack for many occasions. The general recommendations for the spices will help you to get started. However, this recipe encourages you to try your own favorite spice combinations or create new ones too. May the crunch be with you! Prep time: 10 to 15 minutes. Two tortillas make up to 24 pieces.

Ingredients: Organic, local or seasonal
Ezekiel sprouted grain tortillas – 2, (10" size, from frozen foods area)
Olive oil or extra virgin coconut oil, or grapeseed – 1 tsp. (for every 2 tortillas)
Sea salt – sprinkled evenly over top
Thyme leaves - sprinkled evenly over top
Garlic powder - sprinkled evenly over top
Rosemary leaves or powder – a few dashes

Optional:
Cayenne powder – a pinch or two
Herbs de Provence - a pinch or two
Oregano leaves – a pinch or two
Italian spices – a pinch or two

Utensils: Chef's knife or pizza cutter, cutting board, teaspoon, baking sheet, serving bowl.

Directions:
- Preheat the oven to 325.
- On a cutting board, pour 1 tsp. olive oil onto one of the tortillas.
- Take a fresh tortilla and rub it together with the oiled one to coat both tortillas evenly.
- Sprinkle on each of the seasonings.
- Using a chef's knife or pizza cutter, stack the tortillas together evenly and cut them into triangles. To do so, slice the tortillas in half, stack them evenly, and slice in half again. Lastly, carefully stack and cut the sections into thirds to form even-sized triangles.

Baking:
- Arrange the triangles in a single layer on large baking sheet and place in the oven at 325.
- Bake for 12 to 15 minutes, check them periodically, and remove when golden brown.

- Test a crunchy for crunchiness and color.
- Remove them from oven and let cool.

Serving:
Place in a serving bowl and serve alone as a simple snack or along with some 'Chunky Mango Salsa' or 'Whole–You–Guacamole' or 'Simply Tomato Soup'.

Crunchy Roasted Bonzo's

If you're looking for a terrific savory, crunchy snack that's new and different, this recipe fits the menu. With about 15 grams of protein, nearly 13 grams of fiber, less than 300 calories, and notable amounts of folate, iron, magnesium, and potassium, per cup cooked, garbanzo beans may be the perfect low-calorie choice for snacking. They make a great travel snack or something to help you snack through the day in a better way. Try the different variations below and have fun enjoying (and sharing) the tasty results.
Prep time: 40 to 45 minutes.

Ingredients: Organic, local or seasonal
Garbanzo beans – 2, 16oz. cans, drained or 2 cups cooked*
Wheat–free tamari – 2 to 3 Tbsps.,

Optional:
Cayenne pepper – 1 pinch

Utensils: Colander, measuring spoons, mixing bowl, large non-stick sheet, long spoon or rubber spatula.

Directions:
- Pre-heat the oven to 375.
- Rinse and drain the canned garbanzos in a colander.
- Pour them into the mixing bowl, add in the tamari and mix well with a spoon or spatula.
- Assemble the contents on a baking sheet place in the oven. After about 20 minutes, use the spatula to turn the garbanzos to promote even cooking.
- Bake them for another 20 to 25 minutes or until they turn dark brown and have a slight crunch. As they cool, they will become crispier. Total baking time is about 40 to 45 minutes.
- Serve as is, toss them over a mixed greens salad, or add them into a soup.

Variations:
1. Toss the garbanzos in a mixture of 1 Tbsp. virgin olive oil, 1 tsp. of sea salt, 1 tsp. of garlic powder, and a few dashes of cumin and bake as above.
2. For a more savory flavor, toss them in 1 Tbsp., olive oil and a tsp. or two of your favorite curry powder, and bake as above.
3. For a sweeter version, toss them in a light coating of warm raw honey or maple syrup, sprinkle with cinnamon or shredded coconut, and bake for a nice sweet treat.

*Directions for cooking garbanzos at home

- In a large, covered saucepan or large bowl filled ¾ of the way with water, add 1 tsp. of sea salt or a few 1" strips of kombu (sea vegetable) and soak 2 cups of garbanzo beans overnight or at least 6 to 8 hours. It can also be refrigerated.
- The next day, simmer on low heat and add 1 tsp. sea salt. Cooking time is about 2½ to 3 hours.

Tip: The same soaking water can be used for the cooking the garbanzos as well.

- Drain and rinse them in a colander. The finished beans should have a soft and squishy texture.
- Refrigerate in a sealed container and use them within 5 days.

Add Your Own Recipe Ideas Here:

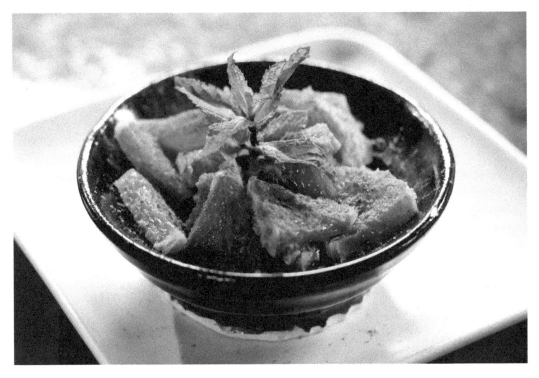

Get in the Groove Grapefruit Breakfast

Get in the Groove Grapefruit Breakfast

If you are looking for a simple, fast, on-the-go, satisfying breakfast addition or snack, this quick recipe is the answer. Grapefruits are a significant source of vitamin C and bioflavinoids, potassium, antioxidants, water, and fiber. By simply sprinkling on the flax or chia seeds, you are increasing your intake of good fiber, protein, and omega 3's for the day. Prep time: 5 to 10 minutes. Serves 1 to 2.

Ingredients: Organic, local or seasonal
Grapefruit - 1 ruby red or pink (Texas Rio or Florida, California, etc.), rinsed
Flaxseed meal or chia seed meal – 1 tsp., (freshly ground if available)
Cinnamon – 1/8 to 1/4 tsp.

Optional:
Shredded coconut – 1 tsp. for garnish
Mint leaves – 2 to 3, rough chopped and sprinkled for garnish

Utensils:
Chef's knife or serrated knife, cutting board, serving bowl, and measuring spoons.

Directions:
- Rinse the grapefruit.
- While peeling off the skin, try to keep some of the white rind attached to the fruit. There's some beneficial fibers contained in the white rind.
- Slice the grapefruit into quarters.
- Cut each piece in half (long ways), lay the pieces on their side and slice across 3 or 4 times to form even, bite-sized, triangles.
- Place the grapefruit pieces into a serving bowl and sprinkle on the flaxseed meal and cinnamon.
- Garnish with any of the desired optional ingredients and serve chilled.

Tip: For a more colorful presentation, try adding in a few slices of blood orange or mandarin oranges.

Michael's Yummy Groats

A simple and appetizing way to expand your breakfast options, buckwheat groats are a practical, gluten-free alternative to the usual breakfast grains. They provide a quality source of protein, sufficient amounts of fiber, magnesium, are slightly alkaline forming, and when cooked, are quite similar in texture to oatmeal. Prep time: 20 to 25 minutes. Serves 2 to 4.

Ingredients: Organic, local or seasonal
Buckwheat groats - 1 cup
Coconut oil – 1 Tbsp.
Sea salt – 1 tsp.
Cinnamon - ½ tsp.
Almond milk – ½ cup
Stevia powder – ¼ tsp., or raw agave nectar or pure maple syrup (warmed) - 2 tsp.
Vanilla extract – 1 tsp.

Optional toppings:
Flaxseed meal – 1 tsp.
Fresh blueberries – as desired
Chopped pecans or walnuts – as desired
Raw cacao powder – 1 Tbsp.
Protein powder – 1 scoop 'Vega One' or favorite plant based protein powder

Utensils: Two quart saucepan, measuring spoons, measuring cup, mixing spoon, and small bowls for any toppings.

Directions:
- Measure the buckwheat groats and bring 2 cups water to a boil.
- Stir in the groats, a pinch of sea salt, coconut oil, and simmer on low heat until all water evaporates (about 15 minutes).
- Before serving, mix in the almond milk, sweetener, vanilla extract and cinnamon.
- Garnish with any of the optional toppings and serve warm.

When you try Michael's Yummy Groats, it's definitely **not** a groat-free zone!

"On the Go"
Quick and Simple Snack ideas

Here are some quick and simple ideas for busy individuals or parents interested in finding more healthy and appetizing options for themselves or their children.

Ingredients: Organic, local or seasonal

1. Fresh or frozen sliced bananas dipped in flaxseed meal sprinkled with cinnamon.
2. Fresh or frozen sliced bananas dipped in raw almond butter or topped with raw cacao (chocolate) nibs.
3. Apples or celery dipped in raw almond butter, sprinkled with flaxseed meal, and a few dashes of cinnamon or shredded coconut flakes.
4. Fruit smoothies – 2 cups filtered water, coconut water, or unsweetened apple juice, 1 or 2 handfuls of frozen organic berries, dash of stevia powder or raw honey, a dash or two of cinnamon, and ice cubes.
5. Homemade or from the store bulk aisle - energy mix a handful each of the following: raw walnuts, dried cranberries (apple juice sweetened), unsalted sunflower seeds, pumpkin seeds, raw almonds, dried coconut pieces, goji berries, sea salt.
6. Fresh or pre-cut, organic fruits and vegetables from the market.
7. Easy wraps – lightly steamed Ezekiel tortilla (insert a colander into saucepan with boiling water, steam tortilla for 10 seconds). Wrap it with fresh sprouts, avocado, tomato slices, a squeeze of lemon or lime juice, a tsp. of extra virgin olive oil or flax oil and a dash of sea salt.

Raw nutrition bar companies online or from the health food store:

Earthling Organics – Earthlingorganics.com, Gopals health snacks – Gopalshealthfoods.com, Go Raw snacks – Goraw.com, Himalania raw food snacks – Himalania.com, Prana bars – Pranabars.com, Vega nutrition bars – Sequelnaturals.com, Wild Bar – Ancientsunnutrition.com

Other simple ideas

Hummus w/ "Crunchies" or carrot sticks.
"Chunky Mango Salsa'" with "Crunchies" or cucumber slices.
"Whole–U–Guacamole" with "Crunchies" or celery sticks.
"Toasted A. B. & J." – raw almond butter and organic jelly sandwich on Ezekiel bread toasted in the skillet.
"Sweet Crunchies Cereal" with "Chocolate Almond Milk" or coconut milk.

Sweet Crunchies Cereal

It's nice to make the morning a little sweeter and crunchier with this recipe. For enhanced nutrition, I highly recommend adding in any of the optional toppings. The main idea here is to have more fun making your breakfast and to enjoy the fruits and the fiber of your efforts. Prep time: 20 minutes. Makes about 1¼ cups.

Ingredients: Organic, local or seasonal
Ezekiel Tortillas – 4 tortillas, 10" size (by Food for Life - in frozen food section)
Raw honey – 1 Tbsp. for each tortilla
Cinnamon – sprinkled over the top
Almond milk – regular or chocolate flavored

Optional toppings:
Chopped walnuts, pecans, or almonds – as desired
Flaxseed meal or chia seed meal – 1 tsp.
Sunflower seeds – 1 tsp.
Fresh or frozen berries – ¼ cup
Fresh or frozen sliced bananas – ¼ cup, sliced thin
Cacao nibs – 1 Tbsp., (raw chocolate pieces)

Utensils: Food processor or blender, prep bowls, non-stick baking sheet, cutting board, pastry brush and measuring spoons.

Directions:
- Pre-heat the oven to 350.
- Arrange the tortillas on a cutting board and apply a layer of honey to each with a pastry brush.
- Sprinkle the cinnamon on top and place tortillas on baking sheet.
- Bake in oven for about 20 to 25 minutes and check them periodically. Tortillas are done when they bend up, turn dark brown, and crispy.
- Remove the tortillas from the oven and let cool.
- If you have a food processor, break up the tortillas into a few smaller pieces, place them into food processor and pulse it a few times to chop them into smaller, bite size morsels.
- Garnish with a sprinkle of any of the above toppings, pour in some almond milk, and enjoy.

Tip: You can also try "Sweet Crunchies" alone as a snack or as a garnish for some of your favorite desserts.

Toasted A.B. & J. Sandwich

As someone who really enjoys a good sandwich, I came up with this recipe as a substitute for the much celebrated peanut butter and jelly sandwich. For those that love the 'P.B.J.', the almond butter and jelly sandwich will not disappoint. In fact, those with peanut allergies will appreciate having this new recipe to add to their sandwich arsenal.
Prep time: 10 to 15 minutes. Server 1 to 2.

Ingredients: Organic or local
Ezekiel 4:9 Sprouted grain bread (from frozen foods section) or whole grain loaf
Raw or roasted almond butter – 1½ Tbsps.
Strawberry or mixed berry jelly* – 1½ Tbsps.
Earth Balance natural buttery spread or extra virgin coconut oil – 1 Tbsp.
Cinnamon – a few pinches on each slice

*Look for organic or local brands that use real fruit, natural fruit sweeteners, have no high-fructose corn syrup, and no added sugars or artificial sweeteners.

Optional toppings:
Raw (cacao) chocolate powder or carob powder – ½ tsp. sprinkled on each side
Fresh or frozen sliced bananas – ½ sliced thin

Utensils: Chef's knife, cutting board, nonstick skillet, measuring spoons, flat spatula, and a spreading knife.

Directions:
- If the bread is still frozen, thaw or warm the slices before spreading.
- Spread on the almond butter and the jelly and close the sandwich.
- Spread a light covering of earth balance or coconut oil and a sprinkle of the cinnamon on the outside of each slice.
- In a skillet on medium heat, add 1 Tbsp. earth balance, allow it to melt and place in the sandwich.
- Toast each side until golden brown and crispy (about 4 to 5 minutes).
- Remove it from the skillet, let cool before slicing.
- Garnish with sprinkles of cinnamon or raw chocolate powder if desired.
- On the cutting board, slice diagonally once or twice to make 2 or 4 triangles.
- Let sandwich cool a bit before serving.**

Variation: For a nice cooking variation, toast the sandwich in a panini press or Foreman style grille. For an extra special treat, add in a few slices of fresh or frozen banana before cooking. It makes a great snack for road trips or the picnic basket. It's surely a sandwich Elvis would have said "thank you very much!" for.

**Messy Clothes Warning:

If this sandwich is eaten while too warm, it can have, let's say, sort of a 'messy' effect on clothes. Basically, biting into this sandwich may cause some unintended oozing out of its contents onto your clothes, the floor, furniture, etc. So, it will help to let the sandwich cool down for about 5 to 10 minutes in order to avoid any undesired food accidents. Or, you may opt to wear a fancy bib instead and enjoy making the mess anyway.

Delectable Drinks and Smoothies

Almond Milk

AM Attitude Protein Smoothie

Gourmet Cashew Milk

Green Machine

Raspberry Lemonade

Raw Nog

Rawsome Fruit Smoothie

Almond Milk

Soaking almonds helps to remove enzyme inhibitors, makes them easier to digest, and lightens their flavor and texture. It also enhances the texture and flavor of the finished milk. Aside from being deliciously creamy and dairy-free, home-made almond milk is an excellent source of monounsaturated fats, minerals like calcium and magnesium, and provides better overall nutrition than store bought varieties. If you try some of the variations, you will find it worth making quite often. Prep time: 10 to 15 minutes.
Makes 1 about quart.

Ingredients: Organic, local or seasonal
Raw almonds – 1 cup (raw variety), soaked overnight
Filtered water – 3½ cups (28 oz.)
Pure vanilla extract – 1 tsp.
Sea salt – one or two dashes
Stevia leaf powder ¼ tsp. or raw agave nectar – 1 Tbsp.

Optional Sweeteners:
Xylitol – 2 tsp.
Coconut palm sugar – 2 or 3.

Variations
Use the same directions as below and mix in these new flavors after blending the original milk.

Strawberry almond milk:
Fresh or frozen organic strawberries – 1 dozen, average-sized
To finish, filter at least once or twice through a fine mesh strainer or cheese cloth.

Chocolate almond Milk:
Raw cacao (chocolate) powder – 2 to 3 Tbsps.

Utensils: Chef's knife, cutting board, hi-speed blender or Vita-mix, large bowl to filter almond milk, glass container or mason jar for storage, measuring spoons, measuring cups, fine mesh strainer, cheese cloth or nut milk bag*.

Directions:
- Pre-soak the almonds in the refrigerator for 6 to 8 hours or overnight.
- Rinse and drain the almonds in the fine mesh strainer.
- Measure the water in the blender.

- Add in the almonds, blend on high speed for 1 to 2 minutes or until well-combined.
- Secure the mesh strainer over a large bowl. Pour in the blender contents and carefully press the liquid through with a soup ladle or large spoon until the liquid stops dripping and pulp looks dry. Save the leftover pulp** if desired.
- Filter contents again back into the blender and blend in all flavorings.
- Taste and adjust the flavor as desired.
- Served chilled with "Sweet Crunchies Cereal" or use it to make your favorite smoothie.
- Refrigerate in a glass mason jar and use within 3 to 4 days.

*Tip: Ordered from the internet (Amazon.com, etc.), a nut milk bag is a more efficient, time-saving way to make nut milk and does not require peeling any almonds. After blending the almonds, simply pour all the contents through the milk bag into a large bowl or Mason jar. Close the bag and carefully squeeze out all of the remaining liquid until finished. Mix in flavorings and finish as above.

**Tip: The leftover almond pulp can be saved for adding extra fiber to a fruit smoothie or dried in a dehydrator to make almond meal flour for gluten-free baking.

AM Attitude Protein Smoothie

This easy-to-prepare meal in a blender helps you make a great start in the morning and provides energy to keep you going all day. It was inspired by my clients' need for a timely, nutrient-dense, and satisfying breakfast. By adding in some of the optional ingredients, this deliciously satisfying recipe helps to curb food cravings, increases energy, aids in muscle repair and growth, promotes weight-loss, supports healthy hair, skin, nails, and improves libido. Having a smoothie like this into your daily routine is a great way to start each day with the right attitude. Prep time 5 to 10 minutes. Makes 3 to 4 cups.

Ingredients: Organic, local or seasonal
Filtered water – 3 cups or (1½ cups water, 1½ cups almond milk)
Protein powder – 1 scoop 'Vega One' or plant-based protein powder
Raw almond butter – 1 Tbsp.
Fresh or frozen berry mix – 1 cup (blueberries, raspberries, blackberries, etc.)
Sliced banana – ½, rough chopped (fresh or frozen)
Sea salt - a few dashes
Ice cubes – 1 or 2 handfuls

Optional:
Flaxseed oil or E.F.A. oil blend – 1 Tbsp.
Maca root powder – 1 Tbsp. (roasted or gelatinized variety – if available)
Ginger root – 1" piece, minced
Ground cinnamon – 1/8 tsp.
Antioxidant drink mix powder – 1 scoop (i.e. acai berry powder or Superior Reds)

Utensils: Chef's knife, cutting board, paring knife, avocado scooper or teaspoon, measuring spoons, blender, measuring cup, chilled serving mugs.

Directions:
- In a blender, add water, protein powder and mix on low for about 30 seconds. Add in the remaining ingredients and mix on high speed for about 1 minute.
- Blend for 1 to 2 minutes on high until very smooth and serve.
- Blend in a few ice cubes if desired.

Tip: If you feel the smoothie alone was not satisfying enough, it's a good idea to eat a small salad, an organic apple or raw food bar afterward. This will give you something to chew on and satisfy cravings until your next major meal.

Gourmet Cashew Milk

In a few minutes, you can make this rich, flavorful, non-dairy beverage that can be used as a substitute in many recipes. Try it with your favorite breakfast cereal, a smoothie, or sauce. This versatile beverage contains good sources of important nutrients like protein, monounsaturated fats, folate, potassium, magnesium, phosphorus, and zinc.
Prep time: 10 minutes. Makes one quart.

Ingredients: Organic, local or seasonal
Raw organic cashews - 3 large handfuls
Filtered water – 2½ cups
Fresh young coconut – 1, (from health foods store) use the meat and water
Ginger root - 1" piece, minced
Medjool dates - 2 or 3, pitted, and rough chopped
Cinnamon – ¼ tsp.
Cardamom powder – a few dashes
Sea salt – a few dashes
Vanilla extract – 1 tsp.

Optional:
Stevia powder – 1/8 tsp. or raw agave nectar - 1 Tbsp.
Coconut milk – ½ cup

Utensils: Chef's knife, cutting board, blender or Vita-mix, measuring spoons, measuring cups, peeler, prep bowls, large sturdy spoon for scooping coconut meat, cheese cloth or mesh strainer.

Directions:
- Measure water in the blender.
- Prepare dates and ginger root as above and place in small prep bowls.
- Open the young coconut with chef's knife, collect the water, scoop out coconut meat, rough chop the meat, and put it into a prep bowl.
- Add in the coconut water, half the coconut meat, cashews, and all other ingredients.
- Blend on high for about 2 minutes or until smooth and creamy.
- If desired, blend in a handful of ice cubes. Taste and adjust flavor and thickness as needed.
- Serve chilled and enjoy!

Note: For a smoother texture, filter once or twice through a cheese cloth or a fine mesh strainer.

Tip: For an ultra-rich, more decadent approach to this recipe, blend in a large scoop of vanilla coconut milk ice cream.

Recipe suggestion: If you really enjoy french toast and are looking for a delicious, dairy-free alternative, this recipe works quite well as a batter substitute. Try it with Ezekiel 4:9 sprouted bread or your favorite gluten-free bread.

Green Machine

For true beauty inside and out, this smooth and flavorsome, longevity promoting drink provides lasting energy to keep you going. With its abundance of chlorophyll, fiber, and phytonutrients, it's a simple, sensible way to start or end the day with more raw, alkalizing foods. This recipe was inspired by the pH miracle and the terrific work of Chef Shelley Redford Young. Although it looks rather green, you'll be pleasantly surprised to learn how taste bud friendly it truly is. Prep time: 15 minutes. Makes 3 to 4, 8oz. servings.

Ingredients: Organic, local or seasonal
Filtered water or coconut water – 3½ cups
Lemon or lime – ½, fresh juiced
Cucumber or English cucumber – ½, rough chopped
Avocado – 1 ripe (small), pitted and scooped (if large, use ½)
Spinach or mixed greens – 1 large handful
Ginger root - 1" piece, peeled, and minced
Sea salt – a few dashes
Apple – 1, Granny Smith or Asian pear - 1, rough chopped
Ice cubes – 1 handful (optional)

Optional:
Flaxseed meal – 1 Tbsp. (from health food store or natural food section)
Pomegranate arils (seeds) – 3 to 4 Tbsps., use them in place of apples
Greens powder – 1 Tbsp., organic greens powder from the health food store
Concentrated liquid chlorophyll – 1 tsp. (from the health food store)
Fresh young coconut* - 1, use the meat and water

Utensils: Chef's knife or paring knife, cutting board, hi-speed blender or Vita-mix, measuring spoons, measuring cups, colander, prep bowl, peeler, sturdy spoon, citrus reamer or juicer.

Directions:
- Rinse and prepare the fruits and vegetables as above.
- Measure the water in the blender.
- Add in lemon juice, ginger, cucumber, avocado, leafy greens, apple, any optional ingredients, and blend on high speed for 1 to 2 minutes.
- If desired, add a few ice cubes to give it a nice chill.
- If too thick, simply adjust with more water, blend, and taste.
- Serve in chilled mugs and enjoy.
- Refrigerate leftovers and drink within one day or freeze for later use.

*Opening the young coconut

Place the coconut on its side on a cutting board next to the sink. Place a bowl or large measuring cup in the sink to collect the water. Using a sharpened chef's knife, carefully trim off the white husk (slicing toward the point) while slowly turning the coconut with your free hand in a circle around the point until you see the top. Using the back of the knife, firmly tap the top of shell in a circle until it cracks and you can pull it off by hand. After opening, filter the water through a mesh strainer. Scoop out the contents of the coconut meat with a sturdy spoon, and rough chop it before blending.

Tip: While scooping out the coconut meat, be careful not to scoop out the harder, brown, inner part of the shell. It's very fibrous and difficult for the blender to liquefy.

Storage: If you are not using the opened coconut right away, store the coconut water and the meat in closed containers in the refrigerator. It will store well for two to three days.

If opening the young coconut is not for you, ask the produce person or a chef to open it for you.

Raspberry Lemonade

If you're looking to satisfy your desire for something tart and refreshing, this drink will fulfill that wish quite well. To prepare this recipe, locate a no additive, organic sorbet in the frozen section of the health food store or the natural foods section of the market. What's interesting to note about this easy-to-prepare beverage is its high content of vitamin C, bioflavinoids, potassium, antioxidants, and phytonutrients. It's ready in about 5 minutes, and provides nature's answer to satisfy your thirst in a delicious way.
Prep time: 5 minutes. Makes one quart.

Ingredients: Organic, local or seasonal
Lemons – 3 to 4, freshly juiced
Filtered water – 1 quart
Lemon sorbet – ½ pint (with no artificial sweeteners or flavorings)
Raspberries – 2 handfuls, for garnish

Optional:
Stevia powder – a dash or two
Mint leaves – for garnish
Ice cubes – a handful or two

Utensils: Chef's knife, cutting board, blender or Vita-mix, measuring spoons, measuring cups, citrus reamer or juicer, sturdy spoon or ice cream scooper.

Directions:
- Measure the water in the blender.
- Juice the lemons.
- Pour the lemon juice into blender, scoop in the sorbet, and add in the stevia powder.
- Mix in the blender on low speed, and gradually turn to high speed for about 1 minute.
- Taste and adjust the flavor with additional sorbet if desired.
- Pour into a chilled container, garnish with the fresh raspberries, and let them steep for a few minutes before serving. This will provide time for the drink to change color.
- Serve in a chilled mug and garnish with a few mint leaves.

Raw Nog

I've served this deliciously rich, satisfying, and versatile beverage for many gatherings, and especially for the holidays. Many are surprised by the fact it's dairy-free and full of nutrition. In fact, it's an excellent source of protein, folate, electrolyte minerals, beneficial medium chain fatty acids from coconut, digestive and immune supporting ginger, and makes a great batter substitute for french toast. Prep time: 5 to 10 minutes.
Makes about 1½ quarts.

Ingredients: Organic, local or seasonal
Raw whole cashews - 3 large handfuls
Filtered water – 3 cups
Pitted Medjool dates – 3, chopped small
Coconut milk – ½ cup (Thai Organic, Native Forest, etc.)
Fresh young coconut – 1, use the meat and water
Cinnamon – 1 tsp.
Vanilla extract – 1 tsp.
Ginger root - 1" piece, peeled, and minced
Pumpkin spice powder – ½ tsp.
Sea salt – ¼ tsp.
Stevia powder – 1/8 tsp.
Ice cubes – 6 or as desired

Optional:
Banana – ½, frozen
Nutmeg – a few dashes
Cayenne – 1 or 2 pinches

Utensils: Chef's knife, cutting board, high speed blender or Vita-mix, measuring spoons, measuring cup, peeler, prep bowl, and a large sturdy spoon for scooping.

Directions:
*   Measure the water in the blender.
*   Open the young coconut with a chef's knife, collect the water and scoop out the coconut meat.
*   Add the coconut water to the blender
*   Rough chop the coconut meat and put into a bowl.
*   Peel and mince the ginger root.
*   Remove and discard the date pits and rough chop the dates.

Mixing:

- In the blender on low speed, add the ginger root, all spices, coconut meat, and mix well.
- Add in chopped dates, coconut milk, cashews, a handful (or two) of ice cubes, and blend on high speed for 1 to 2 minutes.
- Taste and adjust flavor and thickness as desired.
- Pour into a chilled mug, garnish with a sprinkle of cinnamon, a pinch of nutmeg, and enjoy.
- For extra smooth texture and more flavor, add in ½ a frozen banana.

Rawsome Fruit Smoothie

In an effort to include a higher percentage of raw foods in your daily food lifestyle, I created this smoothie recipe to make it a lot easier to accomplish. You can start out by making it this way, try adding some of the optional ingredients, and go on to create new and interesting variations on the basic recipe. This satisfying, longevity promoting drink nourishes the body inside and out, and keeps you feeling great for hours.
Prep time: 10 minutes. Makes 3 to 4, 8oz. servings.

Ingredients: Organic, local or seasonal
Filtered water – 3 cups
Organic coconut milk - ½ cup
Ginger root – 1" piece, rough chopped
Spearmint or peppermint leaves – 6 to 8 leaves, rough chopped
Pitted dates – 2, minced
Raw almonds - ½ cup, blanched (or pre-blanched almonds from the store)
Banana – 1, fresh or frozen
Avocado – ½, pitted and scooped
Ground cinnamon – ½ tsp.
Sea salt – ½ tsp.
Stevia – 1/8 tsp.

Optional:
Mixed berries – ½ cup, fresh or frozen variety
Chia seed meal – 1 Tbsp., from ground chia seeds
Maca powder – 1 Tbsp.
Protein powder – 1 scoop 'Vega One' nutrition shake or other plant-based variety
Antioxidant blend powder – 1 scoop

Utensils: Chef's knife, cutting board, paring knife, avocado scooper or spoon, prep bowls, saucepan and water for blanching, measuring spoons, measuring cup, blender, colander, chilled serving mugs.

Directions:
- Bring water to a boil in a saucepan.
- Submerge the almonds for 1 to 2 minutes.
- Drain them in a strainer, let cool and remove the skins.

Tip: To help the skins come off more easily, place the almonds under slow running cool water as you peel them.

Blending:
- Measure the water and coconut milk in the blender.
- Add in the chopped ingredients, fruit, avocado, spices, stevia, optional ingredients, and blend on high speed for 1 to 2 minutes.
- Blend in a few ice cubes if desired.
- Serve in chilled mugs and garnish with fresh mint leaves.

Tempting Toppings and Sauces

Almost Ricotta Cheeze

Banana Coconut Sauce

Blueberry Vinaigrette

Cheesy Pleasy Sauce

Golden Brown Sauce

Tasty Tomato Sauce

Almost Ricotta Cheeze

The first time I prepared this recipe, I was amazed how much it reminded me of real ricotta cheese. Soaking the raw cashews and macadamia nuts helps to create a smooth, creamy texture that melts in your mouth. Prep time: 10 minutes. Makes about one cup.

Ingredients: Organic, local or seasonal
Raw cashews – ½ cup, soaked 2 to 4 hours
Raw macadamia nuts – ½ cup, soaked 2 to 4 hours
Filtered water – ¼ cup (up to ½ cup or more if needed)
Nutritional yeast flakes – 1 Tbsp.
Garlic powder – ½ tsp.
Miso paste – 2 tsp., mellow white variety
Lemon juice – 1½ - 2 Tbsps.

Optional:
Sea salt – ¼ tsp.
Fresh young coconut meat – 3 Tbsps., rough chopped

Utensils: Chef's knife, cutting board, measuring cup and measuring spoons, food processor or blender, colander and flat spatula.

Directions:
- Using separate mixing bowls ½ filled with water, submerge the cashews and macadamias, a few dashes of sea salt and let soak for 2 to 4 hours.
- Drain the soaked nuts in a colander.

Mixing:
- Measure ¼ cup water to the blender.
- Add in all soaked nuts and pulse the blender until the contents are finely chopped.
- While the blender is on low speed, add in the nutritional yeast, lemon juice, miso paste, optional coconut meat, garlic, and increase to high speed for 1 to 2 minutes.
- Blend until the texture is thick, pourable, smooth, and spreads easily.

Tip: If the blender has difficulty mixing the contents, stop it occasionally, and scrape the sides with a spatula to help mixing. The finished product should have a texture and color similar to that of traditional ricotta cheese.

- Taste and adjust thickness with an additional tsp. or 2 of water or lemon juice if needed.

- Empty contents with a spatula and keep refrigerated in a sealed container.
- Use it for "Mostly Raw Lasagna" or as a dip for your favorite veggies or "Crunchies".
- Stores well in the refrigerator for about 7 days.

Serving tip: When preparing dishes using this cheeze, warming it on a low temperature beforehand helps improve consistency for using as a dip, and makes it easier to spread while preparing the "Mostly Raw Lasagna" recipe.

Banana Coconut Sauce

This richly satisfying sauce helps transform an ordinary sweet potato into an extraordinarily sumptuous dessert. It's quite versatile and can be used to garnish many of your raw and cooked dessert recipes. As it provides a good amount of healthy omega-3 fats, fiber, and potassium, you can smile while enjoying this deliciously decadent topping.
Prep time: 5 to 10 minutes. Makes 1½ to 2 cups.

Ingredients: Organic, local or in season
Coconut milk – 1 cup, (Thai Organic, Native Forest, etc.)
Vanilla extract – 2 tsps.
Stevia powder – 1/8 tsp., or use pure maple syrup - 1 Tbsp.
Flaxseed meal – 2 tsp. (finely ground flaxseeds)
Almonds – ½ cup, blanched
Banana – 1, frozen or fresh

Optional:
Cinnamon – ¼ tsp.
Raw cacao (chocolate) powder – 1 Tbsp.

Utensils: Chef's knife, cutting board, measuring cup and spoons, small saucepan with water for blanching, high speed blender, flat spatula, colander, and prep bowls.

Directions:
- Bring 6 cups of water to a boil in a saucepan, add in almonds, and blanch for 1 minute.
- Drain the almonds and let them cool for a few minutes.
- Under slow-running water, peel off, discard the skins, and place the almonds in a prep bowl.
- With the blender on low speed, add in coconut milk, vanilla, cinnamon, stevia, and flaxseed meal.
- Add in the almonds and bananas, blend on high speed until the sauce thickens, and a smooth texture is reached.
- Taste and adjust flavor.
- Refrigerate in a sealed container and finish contents within 3 to 4 days.

Tip: If the finished sauce comes out too thick, add a few ounces of water, blend, and adjust the flavor as desired.

Blueberry Vinaigrette

By simply adding in the antioxidant power of blueberries, you can turn an ordinary salad dressing into a more colorful, nutritious, gourmet dressing. Blueberries contain hundreds of phytochemicals that support the healing ability of the body on many levels. From protecting us from free radical damage which can cause disease and premature aging to adding color and flavor to recipes, blueberries are an excellent choice to include in your daily food lifestyle. Prep time: 5 to 10 minutes. Makes about 1 cup.

Ingredients: Organic, local or seasonal
Extra virgin olive oil – 6 oz.
Raw apple cider vinegar – 2 oz. (Bragg's or raw organic variety)
Fresh blueberries – 1 cup, rinsed
Sea salt – ½ tsp.
White pepper – a dash or two
Raw honey – 1 tsp.
Lemon juice – ½ lemon, fresh squeezed

Optional:
Flaxseed oil – 6oz., in place of olive oil
Stevia powder – a dash or two, xylitol or coconut palm sugar – 1 tsp.
Thyme – ¼ tsp.

Utensils: Blender, measuring cup and spoons, flat spatula, tasting spoon, and a fine wire-mesh strainer or cheesecloth.

Directions:
- Rinse the blueberries, drain, and set aside.
- In the blender on low speed, add the cider vinegar, lemon juice, all spices, and honey, blueberries, and mix for about 1 minute or until well combined.
- While the blender is running, drizzle in the olive oil and mix well on hi-speed for a few seconds.
- Taste and adjust seasonings.
- Chill before serving.

Finishing the dressing:
- To filter the dressing, pour it though the strainer into a mixing bowl and use a soup ladle or large spoon to gently push the dressing through. Repeat once if necessary.

Cheesy Pleasy Sauce

"If it's cheesy, it's pleasy!" Inspired by the clever saying of a great local chef, this delicious, dairy-free, cheesy substitute provides a rich, creamy texture, a flavorful finish to many dishes, and supplies good nutrition. In addition to being a good source of beta carotene, vitamin C, potassium, and magnesium, this versatile cheese-like topping works well atop veggie burgers, crackers, raw vegetables, and, when thinned out with a little olive oil, creates a rich tasting sauce that can be used for other savory dishes. For best results, serve warm. Prep time: 10 minutes. Makes about one cup.

Ingredients: Organic, local or seasonal
Raw cashews – 1½ cups, soaked 2 to 4 hours
Red pepper – 1, cored, seeded and rough chopped
Filtered water – ¼ cup
Nutritional yeast flakes – 1 Tbsp.
Sea salt – 1 tsp.
Lemon juice – 1 Tbsp., fresh squeezed

Optional:
Cayenne pepper – a pinch or two
Extra virgin olive oil – 2 Tbsps., for a richer, creamier texture
Macadamia nuts – 1½ cup, soaked 2 to 4 hours (substituted for the cashews)

Utensils: Chef's knife, cutting board, measuring cup and measuring spoons, hi-speed blender, colander, flat spatula, and stock bowl.

Directions:
- In a large bowl, soak the cashews for two to four hours, and rinse and drain in a colander.
- Rinse and cut the red pepper as above.

Mixing:
- In a hi-speed blender add in the cashews with ¼ cup of water and pulse until finely chopped.
- While blender is on low speed add in the chopped peppers, nutritional yeast, lemon juice, and sea salt. Increase blender to high speed and blend for 2 minutes, or until creamy smooth.
- Taste and adjust the flavor or the thickness with additional water if needed.

- Empty the contents with a spatula and keep refrigerated in a sealed container.

It stores well for up to two weeks. Use it as a spread for wraps, sandwiches, as a dip for parties with vegetable sticks, or on "Crunchies".

Golden Brown Sauce

Most brown sauces in restaurants or purchased from the market are not gluten-free and may have artificial flavorings, preservatives, or colors added. This homemade version is free of these, has a great flavor, texture, and makes a versatile addition to your collection of sauces. With an exceptional flavor and aroma when served over the "Holiday Loaf" or "Cauliflower Mash", you'll find this savory sauce quite useful and appetizing. Prep time: 20 to 25 minutes. Makes about 1 quart.

Ingredients: Organic, local or seasonal
Olive oil – 3 Tbsps.
Yellow onion – 1, rough chopped
Garlic cloves – 2 tsp., minced
Rubbed sage (dried) – 2 tsp.
Thyme leaves (dried) – 2 tsp.
Nutritional yeast – ½ cup
Pamela's gluten-free baking mix or brown rice flower – ½ cup
Sea salt – 1 tsp.
Tamari – ¼ cup
Water or vegetable stock – 3 to 4 cups

Optional:
Coconut milk – ¼ cup, to thicken at the end

Utensils: Chef's Knife, cutting board, mixing bowls, large saucepan, measuring cup and spoons, skillet, rubber spatula, garlic press or chopper, whisk, stock bowl, or compost bin.

Directions:
- Prepare the onions, garlic as above and measure the dry and wet ingredients.
- In a skillet on low heat, combine the nutritional yeast and baking mix and stir occasionally until warm.

Stir-fry:
- In a saucepan on medium heat, add in the olive oil, onions, and stir-fry for 2 minutes.
- Add in the chopped garlic, sea salt, all other spices, and stir for 2 to 3 minutes.
- Whisk in the warmed skillet contents and combine well in the saucepan.

- Continue whisking quickly as you add in the tamari, most of the water, and allow the sauce to come to a simmer and thicken. Taste and adjust seasonings.
- If necessary, adjust the thickness by whisking in more water or for a creamier finish add in the optional coconut milk.
- Keep warm on low heat and serve over the "Holiday Loaf" or "Silky Cauliflower Mash".

Tasty Tomato Sauce

If you like tomato sauce, you'll love the rich tomato flavor of this simple recipe. Although it's slightly different in texture and flavor, it contains the same beneficial nutritional properties as its soup counterpart. This simple menu addition is easy to enjoy on a regular basis and provides a convenient way to increase your daily supply of antioxidants like lycopene; especially if you include the tomato paste. Prep time: 25 minutes. Makes about 1 quart.

Ingredients: Organic, local or in season
Crushed or diced roma tomatoes – 1, 28 oz. can
Yellow onion – 1, small diced
Extra virgin olive oil – 3 Tbsps.
Garlic – 2 large cloves (or 3 small), minced
Fresh or dried oregano leaves – 1 to 2 tsp.
Fresh or dried basil leaves – 1 to 2 tsp.
Sea salt – 1 tsp.
Lemon juice – 2 tsp.
Filtered water – as needed

Optional:
Sun-dried tomatoes – ¼ cup (whole pieces), minced
Tomato paste – 4 oz. can, half a can

Utensils: Chef's knife, cutting board, measuring cups and spoons, large saucepan, and stock bowl.

Sauce Directions:
- In a large saucepan on medium heat, add in the olive oil, diced onions, chopped garlic cloves, (chopped sun-dried tomatoes), oregano, basil, sea salt, and stir occasionally for 3 to 4 minutes.
- Add in the tomato contents and bring to a simmer.
- To finish, stir in the fresh lemon juice, taste, and adjust seasonings if needed.
- Simmer for 20 to 25 minutes and stir in a few ounces of water to adjust the thickness if necessary.
- After cooling, store in a mason jar, refrigerate and finish within 7 days.
- For a thinner, smoother consistency, blend the contents in a high speed blender for 1 minute.

Scrumptious Soups and Stocks

Better Butternut Squash Soup

Blood Orange Carrot Ginger Soup

Bodacious Black Bean Soup

Broccoli Soup

Hearty Hearty Heart Vegetable Bean Soup

Luscious Lentil Soup

Miso Good Soup

Simply Tomato Soup

Summer Tomato Vegetable Soup

Veggie Smart Stock

Better Butternut Squash Soup

From the arrival of the first cool days of fall, the holidays, and throughout the chill of winter this sumptuously satisfying soup has often been one of my favorites to serve. It contains good sources of vitamin A, folate, vitamin C, potassium, dietary fiber, the anti-inflammatory power of ginger root, is delightfully warming to the body, and smooth on the taste buds. Prep time: 30 to 35 minutes. Serves 8 to 10 (6 ounce portions).

Ingredients: Organic, local or seasonal
Vegetable stock – 1 quart
Water – 1 quart
Butternut squash – 3 lbs., peeled, seeded, medium diced (or pre-cut from store)
Yellow onion – 1, small diced
Ginger root – 1" to 2"piece, peeled and minced
Thyme leaves – 1 tsp. (dried)
Extra virgin olive oil – 3 Tbsps.
Raw agave nectar – 1 Tbsp. or substitute with ¼ tsp. stevia powder
Sea salt – 2 tsp.
Organic cinnamon – ½ tsp.
Coconut milk – ½ cup

Optional:
Cayenne powder – a pinch or two
Green apple – small diced for garnish
Nutmeg or pumpkin spice powder – a few dashes

Utensils: Chef's knife, cutting board, large colander, high speed blender or 10 cup food processor, peeler, large skillet, flat spatula, large soup pot or stockpot, large mixing bowl, measuring cup, measuring spoons, slotted spoon, compost bin or stock bowl, and a ladle.

Directions:
- Fill a large soup pot with the stock and water, bring it to a boil, and add a pinch of sea salt.
- Rinse off the squash, slice it across into thirds (or more depending on the length).
- Remove any of the seeds with a large spoon.
- Blanch (boil with the skin on) the large pieces for about 2 to 3 minutes.
- Remove them from the water with large tongs or slotted spoons, and set aside in a colander to cool for a few minutes.

- On the cutting board, peel off the skin, slice into ½"wide pieces, remove any leftover seeds, and medium dice.

Tip: To save time, keep the soup water simmering so you can use it to cook the squash after dicing it.

- Add the diced squash to soup pot, simmer for about 10 minutes, or until a fork easily pierces through.
- Remove the soup pot from heat and save the cooking water.
- To save the cooking water, insert a large colander into a large mixing bowl in the sink, pour in all contents. Lastly, pull out the colander to drain the remaining liquid and separate the water from the squash.

Stir-fry:
- While the squash is cooking, small dice the onions, and mince the ginger root.
- In a skillet on medium heat, add olive oil, onions, and stir-fry for about 2 to 3 minutes.
- Add in minced ginger root, thyme, sea salt, cayenne (optional), and stir until onions are slightly tender (about 3 to 4 minutes). Remove from heat.

Finishing the soup in the blender:
- Pour 2 to 3 cups of the cooking water into the blender, half the skillet contents, and mix until well combined.
- While blender is on low speed, alternate by adding a few large spoonful's of squash with about one cup of the cooking water until about half of the squash has been used.
- Gradually increase blender to hi-speed, add in the agave, sea salt, cinnamon, and blend until smooth.
- When the blender is nearly full, empty contents into soup pot and repeat the above steps.
- To finish, stir in the coconut milk with the soup and taste and adjust flavor as desired.

Serving:
- Ladle the soup into serving bowls, garnish with a few diced apples, and a pinch of cinnamon or nutmeg.

Blood Orange Carrot Ginger Soup

With its ease of preparation, this soup makes for a delicious, nutritious, budget-friendly, and timely option to add to your weekly menu. As many are aware, carrots are high in beta carotene. They are also good sources of folate, potassium, vitamin K, antioxidants, fiber, support healthy colon function, and promote good vision. Adding in the wakame and blood orange juice enhances the nutritional value, adds a beautiful presentation, and a mouth-watering flavor. Prep time: 20 minutes. Serves 6 to 8 (8 ounce portions).

Ingredients: Organic, local or seasonal
Vegetable stock – 1 quart
Water – 1 quart
Carrots – 2 lbs, rinsed, medium diced
Yellow onion – 1, small diced
Blood orange – ½, juiced
Ginger root – 2" piece, peeled and minced
Thyme leaves – fresh or dried, 1 tsp.
Extra virgin olive oil – 3 Tbsps.
Sea salt – 2 tsp.
Pure stevia powder – 1/8 tsp. or coconut palm sugar – 2 tsps.

Optional:
Wakame flakes (seaweed) 1 tsp., soaked and expanded
Cayenne powder – a pinch or 2
Coconut milk – ½ cup

Utensils: Chef's knife, cutting board, large colander, large prep bowl, bowl of water to expand seaweed, blender, peeler, skillet, wooden spoon or flat spatula, large soup pot, measuring cup, measuring spoons, citrus reamer or juicer, compost bin, ladle, stock bowl.

Directions:
- Prepare the vegetables as above.
- If using the optional wakame, set it aside in a bowl of water for a few minutes to expand.
- In a large soup pot, bring the stock and water mixture to a boil.
- Add in chopped carrots and simmer on low for 8 to 10 minutes or until slightly tender.

- Remove the pot from heat.
- In the sink, insert a colander into a mixing large bowl, pour in the contents, drain the carrots, and save the cooking water to finish the soup.
- Juice the blood orange and save in a prep bowl for use at the end.

Stir-fry:
- While the carrots are simmering, add olive oil into a skillet on medium heat, and stir-fry the onions for 2 to 3 minutes.
- Add in the thyme, sea salt, minced ginger root, a pinch or two of optional cayenne, and stir until onions are slightly tender (about 3 to 4 minutes).
- Remove from heat.

Finishing in the blender:
- Pour in 2 to 3 cups of the cooking water, the skillet contents, blood orange juice, stevia, and blend until smooth.
- To finish, alternate between adding in the carrots and cooking water until all of the carrots are used, and the desired thickness is reached. At this point, it's important to keep an eye on how thick or thin you prefer your finished soup.
- If using the wakame, drain it and mix it in at the end to finish the soup.
- Taste and adjust the seasonings as desired.
- Simmer on low heat and serve warm.

Serving:
Ladle into soup bowls and drizzle in a just a few drops of fresh blood orange juice for a more eye-catching presentation.

Tip: If the soup comes out too thick, add in ½ to 1 cup additional cooking water and mix to desired thickness. Taste and re-adjust seasonings. For a creamier consistency, try finishing the soup with the optional coconut milk.

Add Your Own Recipe Ideas Here:

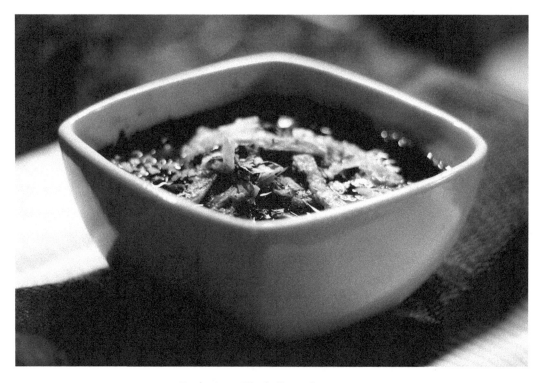

Bodacious Black Bean Soup

Bodacious Black Bean Soup

This soup is a complete meal in one course. If you are looking for a hearty dish that satisfies a hungry appetite, this soup does the job quite well. It has a wonderful array of colors, flavors, and textures. It also provides an excellent source of complete protein, healthy complex carbohydrates, vitamin A, magnesium, iron, and fabulous fiber. You will especially enjoy serving it with baked sweets and "Crunchies" too. Prep time: 35 to 40 minutes. Makes about 3½ quarts.

Ingredients: Organic, local or seasonal
Vegetable broth – 1 quart
Water – 1 quart
Extra virgin olive oil – 3 Tbsps.
Yellow onion – 1, rough chopped
Green pepper – 1, seeded, rough chopped
Red pepper – 1, seeded, rough chopped
Carrots – 1, rough chopped
Broccoli – ½ cup, tops only
Jalapeno pepper – 2, seeded and rough chopped small
Sweet potato – 1, small sized, medium diced
Chili powder - 2 Tbsps.
Cumin powder – 2 tsp.
Sea salt – 2 tsp.
Fresh squeezed lime – ½ lime
Canned diced tomatoes – 1, or use 4 ripe plum or roma tomatoes*
Black beans – 2, 16 oz. cans, drained
Cilantro – 2 Tbsps., rough chopped, for garnish

Optional:
Ezekiel 4:9 corn tortillas** (frozen food section) – 2, baked, sliced into 1" long and thin strips for garnish
Cayenne powder – a few dashes
Frozen organic corn kernels – ½ cup

Utensils: Chef's knife, paring knife, cutting board, large soup pot, saucepan measuring cup and spoons, slotted spoon, baking sheet, citrus reamer or juicer, prep bowls, flat spatula, and stock bowl.

Directions:
- Rinse produce, chop all vegetables as above and place in prep bowls.

Stir-Fry:
- In a soup pot, on medium heat, add olive oil, onions and stir-fry for 2 minutes.
- Mix in the remaining vegetables, all spices, lime juice and stir-fry for 2 minutes.
- Pour in the vegetable broth, water, black beans, diced tomatoes, sweet potatoes, and stir together.

Finishing:
- To finish, stir in an additional 2 Tbsps. chili powder, 1 tsp. cumin, 1 tsp. sea salt, and let simmer for about 20 minutes.
- Taste and adjust flavor with sea salt, chili powder or add in a few dashes of cayenne if desired.
- Before serving, garnish with the tortilla strips, and fresh chopped cilantro.

*If using your own tomatoes:
- In a sauce pan half-full of water, bring it to a boil.
- Slice a small 'X' through the tomato skin on two sides and submerge them for about 1 minute. Remove them with a slotted spoon and let cool.
- Using a paring knife, peel off the skin, core and remove the seeds, rough chop and add them into the soup.

**Making the tortilla strips:
- Preheat the oven to 300.
- On a cutting board, slice tortillas in half, layer them, and cut into 1" long ½" wide strips.
- Arrange them in a single layer on a baking sheet sprinkle with sea salt, a few dashes of black pepper and bake until golden brown (about 10 to 12 minutes).

Add Your Own Recipe Ideas Here:

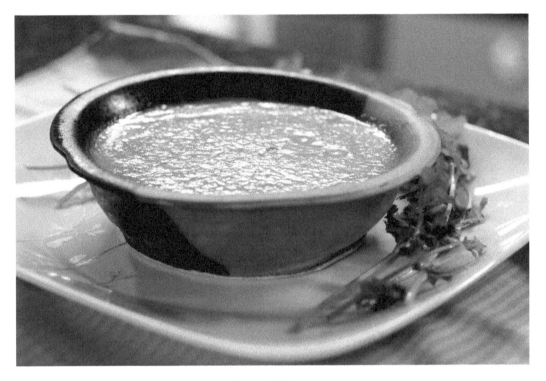

Broccoli Soup

Broccoli Soup

For its simplicity, rich texture, deep flavor, and value, it's hard to beat the convenience of this soup. At around 3 grams per 3 ounce serving (uncooked), broccoli is an excellent source of protein. It also contains noteworthy amounts of vitamin C, vitamin K, folate, magnesium, potassium, phosphorus, and generous amounts of fiber. With great flavor, nutrition and ease of preparation, this soup makes choosing the 'soup du jour' much easier. Prep time: 15 to 20 minutes. Makes about 2 quarts.

Ingredients: Organic, local or seasonal
Vegetable stock – 1 quart
Filtered water – 1 quart
Broccoli – 1 large head, rough chopped into small, bite-sized pieces
Yellow onion – 1, medium diced
Thyme – 1 tsp. (dried)
E.V. olive oil – 3 Tbsps.
Sea salt – 2 tsp.
Coriander seed – 2 tsp., freshly ground
White pepper – ¼ tsp.
Avocado – ½, ripe, pitted and scooped

Utensils: Chef's knife, cutting board, skillet, measuring cup and spoons, large colander, large soup or stockpot colander, food processor and/or blender, mixing bowls, flat spatula, soup ladle, and stock bowl.

Directions:
- Rinse and drain the broccoli.
- Pour the vegetable stock and water into soup pot, and bring it to a simmer.
- Mix in 1 teaspoon sea salt and 1 tsp. coriander.
- While the stock is cooking, cut the vegetables as above.
- Add in the broccoli, cook for 2 to 3 minutes or until slightly tender, and most of the color remains. Remove the pot from heat.
- In the sink, insert the colander into the mixing bowl.
- Pour the soup pot contents into the colander and pull out the colander (separating broccoli from broth).
- Run cold water over the broccoli to stop the cooking process.
- Save the broth for finishing the soup.

Stir-Fry:
- In a skillet on medium heat, add olive oil, onions, all spices, and stir-fry for 3 to 4 minutes.
- Taste and adjust the seasonings and remove from heat.

Finishing in the blender*:
- Spoon half the skillet contents into blender and, using a measuring cup, add 2 to 3 cups of the broth, and blend until smooth.
- With the blender on low speed, gradually spoon in half the broccoli contents, half an avocado and bring the blender to high speed.
- Mix until smooth and adjust the thickness with additional broth if desired.
- Pour blender contents into the soup pot and repeat as above for the remainder of broth, broccoli, and avocado.
- Taste and adjust flavor as desired.
- Serve warm and top with a few pieces of chopped avocado or chopped fresh Italian parsley for garnish.

*Caution – In order to avoid over-filling smaller blender cups, fill it about ¾ full and use two blender cups to finish up the remaining broccoli and broth. If using a Vita-mix blender or a 64 oz. size blender cup, it can all be mixed in one batch. The finished soup should be smooth, creamy and a bright shade of green.

Hearty Hearty Heart Vegetable Bean Soup

If you pick up a package of pre-cut vegetables from the market and some organic canned beans, this heart healthy soup becomes much easier and quicker to prepare. It also provides lots of heart healthy fiber, generous amounts of friendly folate, protein, great flavor, and makes for a satisfying meal. You can add this recipe to your list of spur of the moment meals or for those times you want to make something extra special to warm your heart. Prep time: 30 minutes. Makes about 2½ quarts.

Tip: To save prep time, find a package of pre-cut, fresh or frozen mixed vegetables when available from the produce area or frozen foods section.

Ingredients: Organic, local or seasonal
Extra virgin olive oil – 2 Tbsps.
Carrots - 2, sliced into ¼" half moons
Sweet onion – 1 large, rough chopped
Sea salt – 2 tsp.
Thyme – 2 tsp.
Black pepper – ½ tsp.
Garlic powder – 2 tsp.
Basil leaves – 2 tsp.
Coriander seed powder – 1 tsp.
Vegetable broth – 1 quart
Filtered water – 1½ quarts
Yellow squash – ½, sliced into ¼" half moons
Zucchini – ½, sliced into ¼" half moons
Cauliflower – ½ medium size head, tops cut into bite sized pieces
Broccoli tops – 1 medium size head, cut into bite sized pieces
Great Northern beans or kidney beans – 1, organic 16oz. can
Green peas – 1 cup, fresh or frozen
Lima beans – 1 cup, rinsed and drained, organic variety

Optional:
Green onions – rough chopped and sprinkled for garnish
Bay leaves – 3 or 4
Turnips – 2 small, peeled, medium diced

Utensils: Chef's knife, cutting board, measuring spoons, measuring cup, peeler, colander, large soup pot, wooden spoon or flat spatula, skillet, can opener, ladle, and stock bowl.

Directions:
- Rinse and drain the vegetables, and prepare them as above.

Stir-fry:
- In a soup pot on medium heat, add the olive oil, onions, carrots, spices, and stir-fry for 3 to 4 minutes.
- Pour in the broth, water, all the other vegetables, beans, and stir well.

Finishing:
- Simmer the soup for 20 to 25 minutes and stir occasionally.
- Taste and adjust the seasonings as desired.
- Serve warm with a sprinkle or two of chopped green onion for garnish.

Tip: If you don't have time to do the sir-fry step, skip it and simply pour in all the pre-cut vegetables, beans and spices into the broth right away, stir occasionally, and simmer for 15 to 20 minutes.

Luscious Lentil Soup

This wonderfully delicious and satisfying soup delivers a lot of flavor, is low in calories and, if you have leftovers, is convenient for your next lunch. The coriander seed powder is an important key to the delicate and delicious flavor of this soup and, in addition to its use as culinary spice, contains high amounts of phytonutrients and helps support healthy blood sugar and cholesterol levels. Lentils are an excellent source of protein (18 grams per cup cooked), folate, iron, potassium, important trace minerals, copious amounts of good fiber, and promote healthy cholesterol levels. Prep time: 45 minutes. Makes 2 quarts.

Ingredients: Organic, local or seasonal
Green lentils – 1 cup, rinsed
Vegetable stock – 1 quart (32oz.)
Filtered water – 1½ quarts
Leeks – 1 small bunch, washed and rinsed, rough chopped small
Yellow onion – 1, medium diced
Carrots – 1, sliced into ¼" wide, half moons
Sweet potato – 1, peeled, medium diced
Thyme – 1 tsp. (dried or fresh)
Extra virgin olive oil – 3 Tbsps.
Sea salt – 2 tsp.
Coriander seed powder – 1 tsp. for stir-fry, 1 tsp. to finish the soup
White pepper – ½ tsp.

Optional:
Broccoli – 1 small head, rough chopped small, crowns and stems
Organic frozen peas – 1 cup, thawed
Chopped "Crunchies" for garnish

Utensils: Chef's knife, cutting board, measuring cup and spoons, large colander, large soup or stockpot colander, prep bowls, flat spatula, ladle, and stock bowl.

Directions:
- Soak lentils for 5 to 10 minutes, rinse and drain in a colander.
- Combine the vegetable stock and one quart of water in soup pot and bring to a boil.
- Add in the lentils, 1 tsp. of sea salt, coriander, and simmer until the lentils are soft and squishy (approximately 40 to 45 minutes).
- Fill the sink or large bowl with water, rinse off any dirt from the leeks, and drain. Save for the white (root) end for the stock bowl, or compost.
- While the lentils are simmering, cut the vegetables in order as above.

Stir-fry:

- In a skillet on medium heat, add in the olive oil, onions, leeks, carrots, spices, and stir-fry for 3 to 4 minutes.
- Taste, adjust seasonings, and remove from heat.
- Stir in the skillet contents and diced sweet potatoes.
- Taste and adjust the flavor with sea salt and/or coriander (if needed) to finish soup.
- Simmer on a low heat until the lentils are soft and easy to eat.
- Ladle into soup bowls and serve garnished with chopped green onions or "Crunchies".

Miso Good Soup

Widely used for centuries a condiment in many Asian cultures, miso has many outstanding nutritional qualities. It's a versatile flavor enhancer that adds a richer, deeper flavor to many raw or cooked dishes. In addition to its ability to promote healthy digestion, miso supports immune system health, supplies antioxidants, and contains notable amounts of protein, vitamin K, choline, copper, and zinc. A great soup for colder climates, this recipe is an excellent way to get started using this interesting food. Prep time: 20 to 25 minutes. Makes about 1 quart.

Ingredients: Organic, local or seasonal
Water or vegetable stock – 1 quart
Bok Choy or baby Bok Choy – 2 or 3 full stalks, rough chopped small
Green onions – ½ cup, rough chopped small
Firm tofu – ½ pkg., small diced
Wakame flakes – sea vegetable (from Asian market or health food store) – 1 Tbsp.
Miso – 4 to 5 Tbsps., white or red (soybean paste in refrigerated section).

Utensils: Chef's knife, cutting board, large saucepan, colander, large bowl with water to soak the seaweed, measuring cup, ladle, and stock bowl.

Directions:
- Rinse and drain all the vegetables.
- In a soup pot on medium heat, warm up the water.
- Add in the wakame.
- Cut the vegetables as above, dice the tofu, and add them into the soup pot.
- To prepare the miso, scoop 2 to 3 ladles of the heated soup broth into a measuring cup.
- Spoon in the miso paste and stir until it dissolves and changes the color of the broth.
- Stir the contents back into the soup pot.
- Simmer the soup on low heat for 10 to 15 minutes.
- Ladle into soup bowls, garnish with a sprinkle of chopped green onions, and serve warm.

Simply Tomato Soup

A good friend once told me tomato soup is the soup that heals the soul. Whether you have it warm on a cold day or cool on a hot day, this time-tested, deeply flavorful soup always seems to make the day better. It's so versatile that it can be served alone or with just about any lunch or dinner you can think of. It's no wonder that this was one of the soups I enjoyed most as a little kid and continue loving as a big kid. However, this version has some variations on the original theme. The updated version contains beneficial amounts of Vitamin A, Vitamin K, lycopene, potassium, etc. Prep time: 25 minutes. Makes about 1 quart.

Ingredients: Organic, local or in season
Crushed or diced roma tomatoes – 1, 28 oz. can (fire roasted variety, if available)
Yellow onion – 1, small diced
Sun-dried tomatoes – ¼ cup (whole), soaked and minced
Vegetable broth – 2 cups (divided)
Oregano leaves – fresh or dried, 1 to 2 tsp.
Basil leaves – fresh or dried, 1 to 2 tsp.
White or black pepper – 1/8 tsp.
Sea salt – 1 tsp.
Ripe avocado – ½, pitted and scooped or Earth Balance buttery spread – 1 Tbsp.

Optional:
Chopped parsley – sprinkled for garnish

Utensils: Chef's knife, cutting board, measuring cups and spoons, soaking bowl, soup pot or saucepan, skillet, blender, and stock bowl.

Directions:
- Soak the sun-dried tomatoes in a bowl of warm water for about 10 to 15 minutes or until soft.
- In a large saucepan on medium heat, mix the vegetable broth with the tomato contents and bring to a simmer.
- Mince the sun-dried tomatoes.
- While the tomatoes are simmering, add ¼ cup broth to a skillet on medium heat, add in the diced onions, sun-dried tomatoes, pepper, sea salt, oregano, basil, and stir-fry for 3 to 4 minutes. Remove from heat.
- In a blender, pour in the skillet contents, add 2 cups of the tomato-broth mixture from the soup pot, and blend well.
- To finish, pour the remaining soup pot contents into the blender, add the butter or avocado, and mix on high speed until very smooth.

- Taste and adjust the flavor, thickness, and add extra broth or water if needed.
- Pour the blender contents back into the soup pot and simmer on low heat until ready to serve. Ladle into bowls and sprinkle with fresh parsley for garnish. After cooling, store the soup in a mason jar, refrigerate, and finish within 6 to 7 days.

Summer Tomato Vegetable Soup

On any given day, there are few meals more satisfying than a soup with a sandwich or a wrap. This recipe offers another easy-to-prepare option to include for the daily menu. One of my favorite things about it is versatility. Depending on the season, you can serve it hot or cold and add or subtract any vegetables you desire. Of course, it's best to use as many local, organic, and seasonal vegetables as possible. Prep time: 20 to 25 minutes. Makes 2 quarts.

Ingredients: Organic, local or seasonal
Fresh diced plum tomatoes – 4, or a 28 oz. can diced tomatoes
Vegetable stock or water – 1 quart
Yellow onion – 1 medium diced
Carrots – 1, sliced into ¼" half moons
Lima beans – 1 cup
Broccoli crowns – 1 cup, rough chopped
Basil – 1 Tbsp. (dried or fresh)
Oregano – 1 Tbsp. (dried or fresh)
Extra virgin olive oil – 2 Tbsps.
Sea salt – 2 tsp.
Coriander powder – 1 tsp.
White pepper – ¼ tsp.

Optional:
Fresh basil – small bunch, rough chopped for garnish
Snow peas – ½ cup, rough chopped
Red pepper – 1, medium diced

Utensils: Chef's knife, cutting board, skillet, measuring cup and spoons, large colander, large soup or stockpot, colander, prep bowls, rubber spatula, ladle, and stock bowl.

Directions:
- Rinse and prepare all the vegetables as above and place in prep bowls.
- In a soup pot on medium heat, add in olive oil, onions, carrots, spices, any optional ingredients, and stir-fry for 2 to 3 minutes.
- Add in the vegetable stock, tomatoes into the soup pot, and simmer for 10 to 15 minutes.
- Taste and adjust seasonings.
- Ladle into soup bowls, garnish with chopped fresh basil, and serve.

Veggie Smart Stock

Makes about 2 to 2½ quarts

Ingredients: Organic, local or seasonal
Collected vegetable clippings from the stock bowl – Fill a large bowl with any of the following vegetables: Onions, carrots, broccoli, sweet potato skins, peppers, greens, tomatoes, peppers, celery, cabbage, roots, stems, leaves, and other roots of cut produce, etc.

Use any of the leftover vegetable (only) clippings that you have not used for the recipes you prepared in one week. Make sure the clippings are kept refrigerated in a well-covered or sealed container.

Important: As a general rule, it's best not to keep the stored vegetable clippings for more than one week. However, if not used they will make for good compost.

Utensils: Large stockpot, large colander, large mixing bowl, (2 or 3) quart sized mason jars, large fine wire-mesh strainer or colander, and compost bin.

Directions:
- Fill the stockpot with 2½ to 3 quarts of water (filtered, if available).
- Add the stock bowl clippings to stockpot so they are mostly submerged under water.
- Simmer on low heat for 4 to 5 hours.
- Turn off the heat and let cool for several hours.
- Place a colander inside a large bowl in the sink.
- Pour the contents of stockpot into the colander, lift the colander out of the bowl, squeeze any remaining liquid and discard or compost the cooked vegetable matter.
- Lastly, pour the liquid contents through a fine wire mesh strainer or cheese cloth into glass mason jars to remove any finer particles.
- Seal the jars and refrigerate. The stock will store for up to 2 weeks.
- For longer term storage, make sure to use hard plastic containers or those okay for freezer use.

Satiating Sides

A Taste of Fall

Baked Sweets

High Protein Wheat Berry Salad

Love Your Kale Stir-Fry

Orange-Glazed Tempeh

Quick Jicama Slaw

Rainbow Stir-Fry

Raw Fennel Slaw

Root, Round, Leaf Salad w/ Grapefruit Dressing

Silky Mashed Cauliflower

Steamed Vegetable Supreme

Tri-Color Bliss Potato Salad

Wild Rice Holiday Dressing

A Taste of Fall

This is one of my favorite recipes to prepare as a side dish or dessert for the thanksgiving holidays, or any special occasion. It's full of flavor and has a wonderful aroma that will fill your home with joy. This delicious dish is full of vitamin A, vitamin C, potassium, omega-3's, dietary fiber, and is easy to prepare. Prep time: 45 to 50 minutes. Serves 4 to 6.

Ingredients: Organic, local or seasonal
Sweet potato – 2 large or 3 medium sized, peeled and medium diced
Yellow onion – 1, medium sized, medium diced
Fennel bulb – 1, small (or ½ a large), bulb only, cored, small diced
Green apple – 1 large, cored and sliced into thin wedges
Chopped walnuts – ¾ cup
Dried cranberries – ½ cup (apple juice flavored if available)
Extra virgin olive oil – 2 Tbsps. or vegetable stock - ¼ cup
Maple syrup – ½ cup (pure, no additives variety)
Sea salt – ½ tsp.
Pumpkin spice powder – 2 tsp. (divided)
Cinnamon – 1 tsp.
Extra virgin coconut oil – enough to grease the baking pan

Optional:
Orange zest – 1 Tbsp.
Nutmeg – a few dashes

Utensils: Chef's knife, cutting board, colander, wooden spoon or flat spatula, (2) large mixing bowls, measuring cup, measuring spoons, Pyrex long dish or foil-lined baking sheet, apple corer-divider, peeler, whisk or fork, food service gloves, serving platter, and stock bowl.

Directions:
- Preheat the oven to 350.
- Rinse the sweet potatoes, apples, fennel, and peel the sweet potatoes.
- Prepare the vegetables as above.
- On the cutting board, core and wedge the apple with the apple corer-divider or use a chef's knife.
- Carefully slice each apple wedge in half (long-ways), place the slices on their side, and slice in half.
- In a large mixing bowl, combine the diced sweet potato, onions, fennel, sliced apples, walnuts, and cranberries.

- In a separate mixing bowl, combine the maple syrup with cinnamon, sea salt, 1 tsp. pumpkin spice or cinnamon, any optional ingredients, drizzle in the in olive oil, and whisk well.
- With gloves on or with a rubber spatula, empty the prepared vegetables into the wet mixture, mix, and coat them evenly.

Baking:
- Prepare a foil covered sheet pan or ceramic dish and spread a light coating of coconut oil or natural non-stick spray.
- Assemble the mixture in a single layer, sprinkle ½ tsp. pumpkin spice or cinnamon on top, and bake in oven for about 30 to 35 minutes.*
- Remove and set aside to cool for a few minutes.
- Plate and serve warm.

*While baking, use a spatula or spoon to stir contents periodically. This will ensure even cooking, flavor, and retain moisture. Test the doneness of sweet potato by sticking it gently with a fork. The finished dish should have a soft, chewy texture, and your kitchen will be full of wonderful aromas to enhance the warm, special times in your home.

Baked Sweets

The sweet potato is one of my favorite foods and this recipe is a tribute to its versatility. The benefits of consuming them are quite numerous. In addition to containing high amounts of vitamin A, they are also good sources of vitamin C, antioxidants, manganese, copper, dietary fiber, vitamin B6, potassium, iron, help fight inflammation, and promote blood sugar balance. Try this recipe as side dish with the "Southwest Black Bean Burger" or any veggie burger. Prep time: 40 to 45 minutes. Serves 2 to 4.

Ingredients: Organic, local or seasonal
Sweet potato – 3, medium sized, peeled, medium diced
Olive oil – 2 Tbsps. or vegetable broth – 4 Tbsps.
Sea salt – 2 tsp.
Cumin – 1 tsp.
Chili powder – 1 Tbsp.

Optional:
Cayenne powder – a pinch or two
Garlic clove – 2, rough chopped
Hot sauce – a few dashes of your favorite natural variety

Utensils: Chef's knife, cutting board, large baking sheet pan or casserole dish, large mixing bowl, measuring spoons, colander, prep bowl, peeler, small whisk, flat spatula, and stock bowl.

Directions:
- Preheat the oven to 375.
- Rinse, clean, and peel the sweet potatoes. (If preferred, leave the skin on).
- Medium dice the sweet potatoes.

Dicing Tip: If the sweet potatoes are very large, prepare them as follows:
1. Cut the sweet potatoes in half going across.
2. Cut each piece in half (long ways).
3. Slice each section long ways into ½" wide slices.
4. Lay each piece flat and slice (long ways) to create ½" wide batons or rectangles.
5. Lastly, cube the batons into ½" wide pieces.

Mixing:

- In a mixing bowl, combine the olive oil, all spices, any optional ingredients, and mix well.
- Toss the sweet potatoes in the bowl, and coat them lightly and evenly.

Baking:

- On a foil lined baking sheet lightly coated with coconut oil or non-stick spray, arrange the sweet potato pieces in a single layer, and place them in the oven.
- Bake for 12 minutes, remove from the oven, and turn the sweet potatoes over with a spatula or spoon. Place them back into the oven and repeat this two more times.

Tip: Turning the sweet potatoes each time you check on them prevents sticking and ensures even cooking.

- Test with a fork for doneness and bake a few minutes extra if desired.
- Remove them from the oven and let cool. The finished sweet potatoes should be soft on the inside, light brown and lightly crispy on the outside. The total baking time should be between 35 to 40 minutes.

Serving:

Sprinkle with sea salt and serve warm as a side dish with "Southwest Black Bean Burgers" and "Mango Chunky Salsa".

Add Your Own Recipe Ideas Here:

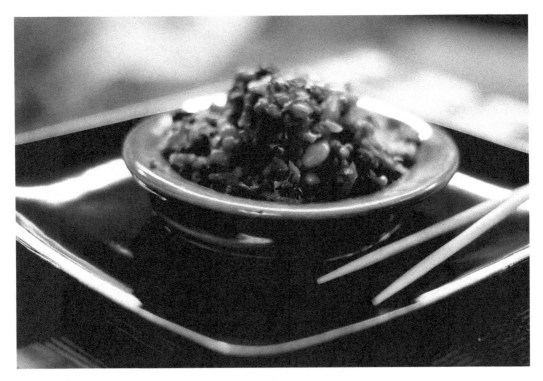

High Protein Wheat Berry Salad

High Protein Wheat Berry Salad

Wheat berries are an excellent source of protein, complex carbohydrates, and fiber. They are a whole, unprocessed, grain that contains all its important components. They also contain a good supply of magnesium, selenium, manganese, and cancer fighting lignans. However, if you know you are very sensitive to wheat or suffer from celiac, it's best to avoid using them and substitute them with lentils, quinoa, or millet. Prep time: 55 to 60 minutes. Serves 2 to 4.

Ingredients: Organic, local or seasonal
Wheat berries – ¾ cup, hard winter, or red winter variety, soaked overnight
Shallots – 2, rough chopped small, or ½ red onion
Sesame oil – 3 Tbsps.
Ginger root – 1" piece, minced
White pepper – 1/8 tsp.
Garlic powder – 1 tsp.
Broccoli tops – 1 cup, chopped small
Carrots – 1 or 2, shredded
Shelled edamame beans (soybeans) – ¾ cup (from frozen foods section)
Dried cranberries – ¼ cup, (apple juice sweetened if available)
Wheat-free tamari – 3 Tbsps.
Lemon juice - 1 Tbsp.
Green onions – rough chopped, sprinkled for garnish

Optional:
Parsley – rough chopped for garnish
Flax oil – 1 Tbsp., for garnish
Mandarin oranges (substitute for the cranberries) – 1, peeled, sectioned

Utensils: Chef's Knife, cutting board, prep bowls, large mixing bowl, large saucepan to soak the wheat berries, colander, measuring cup and spoons, spatula, large skillet, large saucepan, serving platter, spoon, and stock bowl.

Directions:
- In a covered saucepan, soak the wheat berries in 2½ cups water for 6 to 8 hours, or overnight. The same water can be used for cooking them.
- On the stovetop, bring the water to a boil, add in a tsp. of sea salt, and turn down heat to simmer. Cook until most, if not all, the water has evaporated or the kernels expand, and are soft and chewy (about 50 to 55 minutes).

- Remove from heat, drain if necessary, and let cool in a mixing bowl.
- While the wheat berries are cooking, prepare the vegetables as above, and complete the stir-fry.

Stir-Fry:
- In a skillet on medium heat, add in the sesame oil, shallots, and stir-fry for 1 to 2 minutes.
- Add in the minced ginger root, white pepper, garlic, broccoli, shredded carrots, 1 Tbsp. tamari, and stir-fry for 2 to 3 minutes.
- Remove from heat and let cool.

Finishing:
- In a large mixing bowl, add in the thawed edamame, the skillet contents, cranberries,
- 1 to 2 Tbsps. tamari, and lemon juice with the wheat berries, and mix well.
- Taste and adjust the flavor with additional lemon juice or tamari if needed.
- Plate and garnish with a few sprinkles of green onions or chopped parsley.

Love Your Kale Stir-Fry

Kale lovers rejoice! Containing one of the highest nutrient densities per calorie of all fruits and vegetables, this wonderful leafy green food is a smart choice to include lightly cooked or in raw form in a daily smoothie. With the addition of carrots, Brussels sprouts, and fresh garlic cloves, this crunchy-delicious stir-fry is full of great aroma, flavor, nutrition, and a colorful compliment to any meal. A few big pluses of this recipe are its timeliness and ease of preparation, and it's budget friendly. Prep time: 15 to 20 minutes. Serves 2 to 4.

Ingredients: Organic, local or seasonal
Kale – 1 bunch (curly or lacinato), rinsed, de-stemmed, and rough chopped
Yellow onion – 1, medium diced
Carrots – 2 large, sliced into ¼" wide half moons
Brussels sprouts – 2 cups, rinsed, sliced in half, (ends discarded)
Garlic cloves – 6 to 8, rough chopped
Olive oil – 2 to 3 Tbsps. or vegetable stock ¼ cup
Thyme – 1 tsp.
Sea salt – 1 tsp.
Ground pepper – ¼ tsp.
Lemon – 1 Tbsp., freshly juiced

Optional:
Cayenne powder – a few dashes
Lemon zest – 2 or 3 tsps.

Utensils: Chef's knife, cutting board, colander, large skillet, measuring cups and spoons, rubber spatula, zester, and stock bowl.

Directions:
- Rinse and prepare all the vegetables as above.

Stir-Fry:
- In a large skillet on medium heat, add in the oil or stock and sauté the onions for about 2 minutes.
- Stir in the garlic, spices, Brussels, carrots, kale, lemon juice, or optional lemon zest.
- Sauté for 4 to 5 minutes, the kale reduces down, and the vegetables are still crunchy. Remove the skillet from heat.
- Taste and adjust seasonings if desired.
- Plate and serve warm.

Orange-Glazed Tempeh

Tempeh is a highly nutritious food usually made from fermented soybeans. It's typically made by cooking and de-hulling soybeans, introducing a specific type of beneficial bacteria or culturing agent to the soybeans, and then incubating until it forms a solid cake. Its high protein content (20 grams per 4oz. serving) makes it a fitting substitute for meat. Alone, it has a neutral flavor and takes on whatever flavor(s) you use. Prep time: 15 minutes.

Ingredients: Organic, local or seasonal
Tempeh - 16 oz. package – medium diced
Brown rice vinegar – 2/3 cup (from Asian market or international foods section)
Brown rice syrup – 1/3 cup (from the baking section)
Maple syrup – ½ cup
Fresh squeezed orange juice – 1/3 cup (about 1 large orange)
Wheat-free tamari – 1/3 cup (found in Asian section)
Toasted sesame oil – 2 Tbsps. (found in Asian section)
Ginger root – 1 tsp., grated fresh or dried powder
Cumin powder – ½ tsp.
Orange zest – 1 Tbsp. finely grated orange

Utensils: Chef's knife, cutting board, oven proof deep casserole dish for marinating, measuring cups and spoons, large mixing bowl, whisk, zester or boxed shredder, prep bowls, pastry brush, and a flat spatula.

Directions:
- Medium dice the tempeh.
- Prepare the orange zest and measure out the marinate mixture as above.

Marinate:
- Whisk together the vinegar, maple syrup, rice syrup, orange juice, tamari, sesame oil, ginger root, cumin, and orange zest. After whisking the mixture well, pour contents into casserole dish.
- Place the tempeh pieces into the dish, make sure all of them are covered in the liquid, and let marinate for 8 hours or more.

Cooking:
- Preheat the broiler. Line a heavy baking sheet with aluminum foil and spread tempeh in a single layer. Using a pastry brush or spoon, cover the tops of the tempeh pieces with some of the remaining marinade.

- Broil for 2 to 3 minutes only*, turn pieces over with spatula, brush them again, broil for 2 to 3 more minutes or until golden brown, and heated through.
- Remove them from oven immediately and let cool.

*For best results, keep an eye on the tempeh. Experience has taught me that it's very easy to overcook it in the broiler.

Serving and storage:

The finished tempeh is quite versatile and goes great on top of buckwheat soba noodles, udon or Thai noodles, wild rice, brown rice, steamed or stir-fried vegetables, and with green salads. It's best served warm but can be served cold as well. Refrigerate in a sealed container and use within 3 to 4 days.

Quick Jicama Slaw

As a delicious, colorful topping for your favorite salad, sandwich or veggie burger, this slaw adds an extra-special pizzazz to the flavor and presentation of the food on the plate. Jicama is also a great addition to salads or used for dipping into any of your favorite dips. This quick and easy-to-prepare recipe comes with ample amounts of vitamin A, vitamin C, potassium, fiber, water, and is naturally low in calories. Prep time: 10 to 15 minutes. Makes 2 to 4 servings.

Ingredients: Organic, local or seasonal
Jicama – 1 (medium sized), shredded
Corn kernels – 1 cup, fresh or frozen
Cilantro – ¼ cup, rough chopped
Red pepper – ½, small diced
Lime – 1, fresh squeezed
Sea salt – 1 tsp.
Cumin – ¼ tsp.
Apple cider vinegar – 1 Tbsp.

Optional:
Lime zest – 2 tsp.
Cayenne pepper – 1 pinch

Utensils: Chef's knife, cutting board, box shredder or food processor, prep bowls, large mixing bowl, colander, citrus reamer or juicer, measuring spoons, peeler, flat spatula or mixing spoon, zester, and stock bowl.

Directions:
- Rinse and drain all the vegetables.
- Peel the jicama, prepare all vegetables as above, and place in prep bowls.
- Using the large hole on the box shredder or a food processor with shredding blade, shred the jicama, and place contents into a mixing bowl.
- Add in the chopped cilantro, red pepper, corn, lime juice, spices, and mix well with a spatula.
- Taste and adjust seasonings.
- Chill and serve.
- Use as a topping for your favorite salads, tacos, burgers, or main dishes.

Tips on choosing and storing jicama:

Choose jicamas that are solid and firm, have a good shape, color, and no visible mold on the skin. If uncut, store them in the crisper of the refrigerator. If any of the skin has already been peeled off, cover area with a moist paper towel or store peeled and sliced jicama in water in a sealed container to extend freshness. Use stored jicama within a week.

Rainbow Stir-Fry

Use this recipe as a guide and then let your imagination go to make foods using the colors of the rainbow. You'll also find this recipe helpful when you want to finish leftover produce in the fridge. In that case you might call this recipe refrigerator stir-fry. By eating from all the colors of the vegetable rainbow you're also getting great flavors, nutrition, and a beautiful presentation. Prep time: 15 minutes. Serves 4 to 6.

Tip: To save prep time, pick up a package of pre-cut, mixed vegetables when available from the fresh produce area or a frozen no additive, or organic variety.

Ingredients: Organic, local or seasonal
Sweet onion – 1, rough chopped
Garlic cloves – 3, minced
Sea salt – 1 tsp.
Thyme leaves – 1 tsp.
Cumin – 1 tsp.
Carrots – 1, sliced into ¼" wide half moons
Broccoli – ½ cup, crowns, bite-sized pieces
Cauliflower – ½ cup, crowns, bite-sized pieces
Red pepper – 1, julienne (thin, stick-like slices) then cut in half
Yellow squash – 1, medium diced
Lemon juice – ½, fresh juiced
Virgin olive oil – 3 Tbsps. or vegetable stock – ¼ cup

Optional:
Lemon zest – 2 tsp.
Cayenne powder – 1 or 2 dashes

Utensils: Chef's knife, cutting board, measuring cup and measuring spoons, large skillet or wok, prep bowls, colander, flat spatula, citrus reamer or juicer, zester or box shredder, and stock bowl.

Directions:
- Fill the sink or a large bowl with water, rinse the vegetables, and drain in a colander.
- Cut the vegetables as above and place them into prep bowls.

Stir-fry:
- In skillet or wok on medium heat, add in the olive oil, onions and stir-fry for 2 to 3 minutes.

- Mix in the minced garlic, and the spices.
- Add in the remaining vegetables (in the order listed above), lemon juice, and stir contents for 3 to 5 minutes or until slightly tender.
- Taste and adjust seasonings.
- Plate and garnish with lemon zest or a dash or two of cayenne powder if desired.

Raw Fennel Slaw

If you love fennel, you may find this recipe to be a welcome variation on the typical slaw theme. If you have not tried fennel before, you may be pleasantly surprised by the flavor of this recipe. With its very delicate sweetness, light licorice taste, and a bold crunch, fennel makes a great substitute to use in many of your recipes. Fennel is a good source of vitamin C, folate, potassium, calcium, fiber, phytonutrients, supports digestion, intestinal health, is less filling, and tastes great. Prep time: 15 to 20 minutes. Serves 2 to 4.

Ingredients: Organic, local or seasonal
Fennel bulb – 2 small or 1 large, cored, and shredded
Red cabbage – ½ cup, rough chopped small
Carrots – ½ cup, peeled and shredded
Veganaise – 3 to 4 Tbsps. (Vegan mayonnaise variety from the health food store)
Sea salt – ½ tsp.
Celery seed powder – ½ tsp. to 1 tsp.
White pepper – 1/8 tsp.
Cumin – ¼ tsp.
Lemon juice – 3 Tbsps., fresh squeezed
Raw honey – 1 Tbsp. (local variety)

Optional:
Red radishes - 2, shredded
Parsley – rough chopped, for garnish

Utensils: Chef's knife, cutting board, box shredder or food processor with shredding blade, large and small mixing bowl, colander, citrus reamer or juicer, measuring spoons, measuring cup, peeler, flat spatula or mixing spoon, stock bowl.

Directions:
- Rinse and drain all the vegetables.
- Prepare the vegetables as above and mix them together in a large mixing bowl.
- You can also save the fennel leaves for the stock bowl or toss them into a mixed green salad.
- In a mixing bowl, mix together the mayonnaise, lemon juice, spices, and honey.
- Pour the prepared vegetables in with mayonnaise mixture and mix well.

- Taste and adjust flavor if desired.
- Plate and garnish with a sprinkle of chopped parsley or fennel leaves.

Keep it refrigerated in a sealed container and finish within one week.

Root, Round, Leaf Salad with Grapefruit Dressing

For those that have not yet tried beets and jicama (Mexican potato) in this way, you will be pleasantly surprised by the delightful flavors and textures of this dish. It has a nice balance of sweet and savory on the taste buds, a good crunch, and is simple and timely to prepare. However, in case any unintended 'food accidents' happen, it's definitely a good idea to wear an apron and a pair of food service gloves while preparing it. Some interesting nutritional highlights of this recipe include: significant sources of beta carotene, vitamin c, folate, potassium, iron, fiber, phytonutrients like liminoids, and lycopene, etc. Prep time: 25 minutes. Serves 4 to 6.

Ingredients: Organic, local or seasonal
Red beets – 3, small sized, peeled, shredded or sliced into thin strips
Gold beets – 3, small sized, peeled, shredded or sliced into thin strips
Jicama – 1 medium sized, shredded or julienne (thin, stick-like slices)
Fresh basil Leaves – 1 pkg. whole, de-stemmed
Cherry or grape tomatoes – 1 pint, sliced in half

Dressing:
Grapefruit – 1 juiced (Texas Rio or Ruby Red)
Sea salt – 1 tsp.
Black pepper – 1/8 tsp.
Apple cider vinegar (Bragg's or an unfiltered, organic variety) – 1½ Tbsps.
Grapeseed oil or extra virgin olive oil – 2 Tbsps.
Raw honey or raw agave – 1 Tbsp.

Optional:
Grapefruit zest – add as garnish
Fennel Bulb – julienne – ¼ cup
Mandarin orange - 1 separated into wedges

Utensils: Chef's Knife, paring knife, cutting board, prep bowls, colander, measuring cup and spoons, whisk and mixing bowl or a blender, peeler, citrus reamer or juicer, boxed shredder, serving platter and spoon, stock bowl, and a pair of food service gloves and an apron for sure.

Directions:
- Rinse and clean the beets and jicama.
- If you have beet green tops, remove & save them for juicing, a stir-fry, or the stock bowl.
- De-stem the basil and shake them clean if necessary.

- Peel the beets and jicama and shred them over a large mixing bowl.

Tip: Use a pair of food service gloves and an apron for this part.

- Using a paring knife, slice tomatoes in half and add them to the mixing bowl.
- Rough chop the basil leaves and mix them in with the grape tomatoes, beets and jicama.

Dressing:
- Juice the grapefruit.
- In a mixing bowl or large measuring cup whisk together the cider vinegar, raw honey, grapefruit juice, sea salt and pepper and lastly, drizzle in the olive oil, and mix.
- Taste and adjust the flavor if necessary.

Serving:
- Pour the dressing in with the salad contents, toss by hand until moist.
- Garnish with a few sprinkles of grapefruit zest and serve chilled.
- Refrigerate in a sealed container and finish within 4 or 5 days.

Tip: The water content of the vegetables adds more liquid to the salad dressing so mixing in a little less dressing is a good idea. You can always add more later if desired.

Tip: If you have a mandolin slicer, use the julienne blade for the beets and jicama to create more visual appeal.

Silky Cauliflower Mash

Move over mashed potatoes and say hello to mashed cauliflower. Once you try this recipe, you will be surprised how satisfying cauliflower is as a substitute for potatoes. When in season, try the darker colored varieties for a more visual appeal. For those interested in lowering their carbohydrate intake, this is a useful option to make regularly. The finished recipe contains a good source of vitamin C, folate, potassium, selenium, healthy fats, and dietary fiber. Prep time: 20 minutes. Makes about one pint.

Ingredients: Organic, local or seasonal
Cauliflower – 1 medium sized head, (regular or colored variety)
Yellow onion – 1 medium sized, small dice
Thyme – 1 tsp. (dried or fresh)
Extra virgin olive oil – (divided) 3 Tbsps. for the stir-fry, 2 Tbsps. to finish
Sea salt – 2 tsp. (divided) 1 tsp. for stir-fry, 1 tsp. to finish
Rosemary powder – 1 tsp. fresh or dried
Parsley – 1 Tbsp. as garnish, rough chopped

Optional:
Cayenne pepper – 1 or 2 pinches
Chives - 2 Tbsps. for garnish
Coconut milk – 2 Tbsps.

Utensils: Chef's knife, paring knife, cutting board, steamer or colander* inserted into saucepan, large skillet, measuring cup and spoons, colander, prep bowls, food processor or blender, flat spatula, serving bowl, stock bowl, and compost bin.

Directions:
- Rinse and drain cauliflower.
- Turn on the steamer or bring water to a boil in a saucepan with a colander inserted.
- Using a chef's knife or paring knife, prepare the cauliflower by: cutting or pulling off the leaves and then cutting around the stem in a circle to remove it.
- With a chef's knife, slice the cauliflower head crosswise into four equal parts.
- Cut off all cauliflower tops (florets) rough chop and pull them apart by hand into small, bite sized pieces. (Set aside the thickest stem pieces for the stock bowl or compost).

Steaming:
- Place cauliflower into the steamer and cook for about 3 to 4 minutes.
- When finished, immediately remove from heat and rinse in cold water.

Tip: For best results, stir occasionally and check the cauliflower to prevent overcooking. This way it still has most of its flavor, nutrition, and has a light crunch.

*If a steamer is not available, bring a large sauce pan filled with about 1" to 2" of water to a boil, insert a metal colander or wire mesh and cover with a lid. For even cooking, make sure to stir the contents occasionally until done.

Stir-Fry:
- In a skillet on medium heat, add in the olive oil, onions, spices, sea salt, and stir-fry for 3 to 4 minutes.
- Taste, adjust the flavor if necessary, and remove from heat.

Finishing in food processor or blender:
- Using a wooden spoon or flat spatula, empty the skillet contents into the food processor or blend, and mix until smooth.
- Add in the cauliflower, olive oil, sea salt, and pulse several times until the contents are mostly smooth.
- Taste and adjust seasonings.
- Plate and garnish with a sprinkle of parsley or chives.

Tip: For a thicker, chunkier texture, add in less olive oil when mixing at the end, and the pulse food processor to desired thickness. For a smoother, more whipped texture, add 1 or 2 Tbsps. additional of olive oil or coconut milk, and process until smooth and creamy.

Steamed Vegetable Supreme

Steaming is one of the fastest and easiest ways to prepare a nourishing, home cooked meal. You can use this recipe as a guide or substitute any three to four vegetable combinations you wish. Important things to be aware of while cooking are taste, color, and texture. Checking occasionally helps to prevent overcooking, retain more flavor, color, and nutrients. Prep time 15 to 20 minutes. Serves 2 to 4.

Ingredients: Organic, local or seasonal
Brussels sprouts – 2 cups, rinsed, stems removed, and sliced in half
Carrots – 1 large – sliced into ¼" wide half moons
Yellow squash – 1 medium sized, sliced into ¼"half moons
Cauliflower – 1 cup, small crowns
Beets – 1 medium sized, red or gold, rinsed, peeled, and small diced
Sea salt – 1 tsp.
White pepper – 1/8 tsp.
Thyme leaves – 1 tsp.
Garlic powder – 1 tsp.

Optional:
"Cheesy Pleasy Sauce" – for garnish
Sprouted firm tofu* – ½ package, medium diced

Utensils: Chef's knife, cutting board, colander inserted into large saucepan or steamer, large mixing bowl, prep bowls, large wooden spoon or flat spatula, stock bowl.

Directions:
- Rinse and prepare all vegetables as above and combine in a large mixing bowl or colander.

*To prepare the tofu, drain off any excess water by gently pressing it between two small plates before slicing. Dice the tofu and set it aside in a bowl to add to finished vegetables. It can also be baked in the oven until golden brown or used fresh.

- Bring the steamer up to temperature or use a saucepan with 1" to 2" of water to a boil and insert a colander.

Steamer:

- Add in the vegetables and steam for 4 to 5 minutes. Check for color, taste, and crunchiness. To ensure even cooking, stir the vegetables a few times during the cooking process, and check for desired flavor and texture.
- Remove from heat, empty the contents into a large mixing bowl, mix in the spices, and taste.
- Plate, garnish as desired, and serve warm.

Tip: If you do not have enough prep time, check the produce department for pre-cut fresh vegetables or the frozen food section for organic vegetable combinations with no additives or preservatives.

Tri-Color Bliss Potato Salad

Potato salad lovers of the world, this recipe is for you. Growing up, I really enjoyed freshly made potato salad; especially the times my Mom prepared it for holidays, big family gatherings, or summer barbecues. My goal with this recipe is to create a richer tasting, more colorful salad, and enhance it with additional nutritional value. For some extra flavor and omega-3 fats, try adding in a tsp. or two of flaxseed oil. Prep time: 25 to 30 minutes. Serves 2 to 4.

Ingredients: Organic, local or seasonal

Red potatoes, yellow or purple potato, sweet potato – 2 even-sized of each type, medium diced

Red onion – 1 medium sized, rough chopped small

Fennel stalks - 3, small diced, leaves removed

Red pepper – 1, rough chopped small

Cayenne pepper – 2 pinches

Cumin – ¼ tsp.

White pepper – 1/8 tsp.

Lemon – 2 tsp., fresh squeezed

Veganaise – vegan mayonnaise, 'Follow Your Heart' (refrigerated section of health food store) 2 to 3 Tbsps. – regular or grapeseed oil variety

Italian or curly parsley – ¼ cup, rough chopped for garnish

Sea salt – 1 tsp.

Optional:

Flaxseed oil – 2 to 3 tsp., mixed in at the end

Utensils: Chef's knife, cutting board, 6 qt. saucepan, measuring cup and spoons, colander, prep bowls, large mixing bowl, serving platter, flat spatula, and stock bowl.

Directions:

- Rinse, clean, and leave the potato skins on.
- Cut all produce as above.
- Bring 6 quarts water to a boil, add in the potatoes*, and let simmer for 10 to 15 minutes.
- Drain in a colander and let cool.

*Cooking Tip – Potatoes have different cooking rates so add them in the following manner: yellow potatoes first, wait about 4 minutes, red potatoes, wait about 4 minutes, and lastly, add in the purple and sweet potatoes. Cook for 5 to 10 more minutes and test softness with a fork.

Mixing:
- In a large mixing bowl, add in veganaise, lemon juice, and use a spatula to fold in all the chopped vegetables, sea salt, and spices.
- Combine the potatoes with wet mixture and mix well.
- Taste and adjust seasonings as desired.
- Plate, garnish with chopped parsley, and serve.

Wild Rice Holiday Dressing

Although it's more a grass than a true grain, wild rice is an excellent choice for those interested in cutting down on grains, carbohydrates, and is more alkalizing to the body. It contains noteworthy amounts of protein (about 3.5 grams per ½ cup cooked), manganese, potassium and zinc, B vitamins, folic acid, and complex carbohydrates. Many find the nutty flavor and soft, chewy texture quite satisfying and it's one of the reasons this recipe works so well. Total prep time: 90 minutes. Serves 2 to 4.

Ingredients: Organic, local or seasonal
Wild rice – ½ cup
Croutons – 6 slices gluten-free bread, medium diced
Sage leaf powder - 2 tsp.
Rosemary – 1 tsp.
Sea salt – 1 tsp.
Thyme – 1 tsp.
Extra virgin olive oil – 2 Tbsps.
Vegetable broth – ½ cup (self-made or organic brand)
Yellow onion– 1 medium sized, medium diced
Fennel stalks – 2 to 3, rough chopped
Pecans – ¾ cup, rough chopped
Extra virgin coconut oil – 1 tsp.

Utensils: Chef's knife, cutting board, (2) large mixing bowls, measuring cup, sauce pan, measuring spoons, compost bin, large baking sheet, non-stick ceramic or rectangular loaf pan, stock bowl.

Directions:
Tip: To save more time, cook the wild rice the night before and refrigerate in a sealed container.
- Rinse the wild rice, vegetables, and drain.

Wild Rice:
- In a sauce pan, bring 1¼ cups water to a boil, wild rice, a pinch or two of sea salt, coconut oil, and simmer on low for about 50 minutes. Remove from heat. The rice is done when it expands, is soft and slightly chewy, and the water has been absorbed.

Croutons:
- Preheat the oven to 325.
- Dice the bread slices into ½" cubes.

- In a separate bowl, mix olive oil with all above spices, and toss in the bread cubes.
- Arrange the croutons in a single layer on a baking sheet.
- Bake them at 325 for 15 minutes or until golden brown and crunchy.
- Remove them from the oven and let cool.

Stir-Fry:

- In a skillet on medium heat, add in half the vegetable broth and stir-fry the onions, all above spices, chopped fennel stalks for 3 to 4 minutes.
- Remove from heat and let cool.
- In a large mixing bowl, combine skillet contents with the wild rice, pecans, croutons, and mix well.

Tip: Test the mixture for enough moisture. If necessary, add in more vegetable broth. The finished mixture should feel moist and not too soft or mushy.

Baking & Serving

- Pack the contents into a non-stick baking rectangular pan, cover the top with aluminum foil and bake @ 325 for 20 to 25 minutes. Remove the foil and bake an additional 10 to 15 minutes or until the top is golden brown and crispy.
- Remove from oven and let cool.
- Slice into 1" wide pieces, remove with a serving spatula, plate, and serve.
- If desired, garnish with a ladle of "Golden Brown Sauce", green onions, and serve.

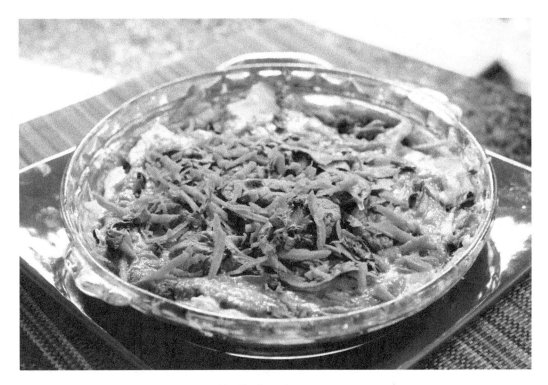

Mostly Raw Lasagna

Enchanting Entrees

Asian Noodle Stir-Fry

Cheesy Red Quinoa

Chickpea Spinach Curry

Holiday Loaf with Brown Sauce

Holiday Quinoa

In No Hurry Curry Lentils

Magic Quinoa

Mama's Millet Chili

Mexican Quinoa

Mostly Raw Lasagna

My Thai Stir-fry

Nori Veggie Wrap

Polenta Lasagna

Simple Tofu Stir-Fry

Soba Florentine

Southwestern Black Bean Burger

Squash Party

Veggie Pizza Quesadilla

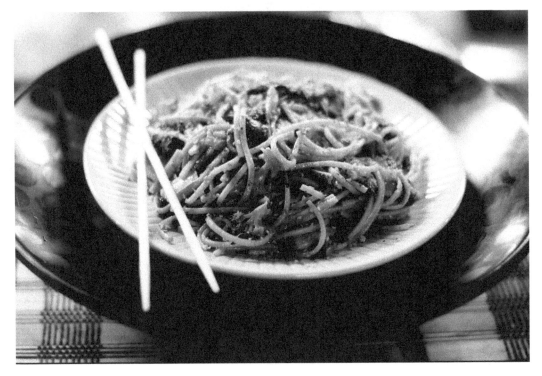

Asian Noodle Stir-Fry

Asian Noodle Stir-Fry

Inspired by the philosophy of macrobiotic cuisine, this aromatic, colorful, and delectable dish has a lot to offer. By adding in the black currants and ginger your taste buds will enjoy the major tastes of the palate. This recipe is low in calories, gluten-free, high in vitamins, trace minerals, plant-based proteins, monounsaturated fats, fiber, and big on flavor. Prep time: 35 to 40 minutes. Serves 4 to 6.

Ingredients: Organic, local or seasonal
Wakame flakes (sea vegetable) – 1 Tbsp., soaked & expanded
Buckwheat soba noodles – 8 oz. pkg.
Edamame beans (shelled soybeans) – 1½ cups, thawed (frozen foods area)
Red & yellow peppers – 1 of each, cored, seeded, 2" long, thin slices
Daikon radish - 2" piece, peeled, julienne
Broccoli – 1 medium crown, tops broken into small pieces
Ginger root – ½" piece, minced
Sesame oil – 4 Tbsps.
Wheat-free tamari – ½ cup, (organic variety, if available)
Gomasio – 2 to 3 Tbsps. (toasted, seasoned sesame seeds in Asian foods area)
Parsley – ½ cup, rough chopped for garnish

Optional:
Organic extra firm tofu* - ½ pkg. (regular or sprouted variety), drained, medium diced
Dried black currants – ½ cup, for garnish

Utensils: Chef's knife, cutting board, colander, prep bowls, spatula or wooden spoon, large mixing bowl, large skillet or wok, large saucepan, measuring cup and measuring spoons, bowl of water for soaking seaweed, colander, peeler, and stock bowl.

Directions:
- Presoak the seaweed in a bowl of water and let it expand for a few minutes.
- Rinse, thaw, and drain all veggies as needed.
- Cut and prepare all vegetables as above.
- *Before dicing, place the tofu between two small plates and press them together gently over the sink to drain off any remaining moisture.

Cooking the soba:
- Bring 6 cups of water to a boil.

- Break the noodles in half, drop in, add a pinch of sea salt, turn heat to low, and simmer.
- Cook for about 5 to 6 minutes or until the noodles are slightly chewy.
- Rinse with cold water, drain, and set aside in a large mixing bowl.

In a skillet or wok:

- On medium heat, warm a large skillet or wok and add in the sesame oil.
- Stir-fry the tofu cubes until golden brown on both sides (8 to 10 minutes per side). Remove the tofu from skillet, and cover to keep warm.
- Add in the ginger root, broccoli, peppers, daikon, edamame, seaweed**, more sesame oil if needed, and stir–fry for 3 to 4 minutes. Remove from heat.
- To finish, combine the skillet contents with soba noodles, tofu, mix in the tamari, and keep warm until serving.

**Drain the seaweed before adding it to the stir-fry.

Serving:

- Plate and garnish by sprinkling on the gomasio, chopped parsley, or optional black currants.

Cheesy Red Quinoa

While experimenting with quinoa, I discovered the delicious flavor of this recipe by accidentally adding in some "Cheesy Pleasy Sauce". It tastes a lot like macaroni and cheese and is a terrific gluten-free substitute. Kids will really enjoy this recipe and it may bring out the kid in you when you try it. Quinoa supplies all the essential amino acids and comes with at least six grams of protein per three ounce serving. It's a good source of magnesium, manganese, iron and fiber, etc. Prep time: 30 to 35 minutes. Serves 2 to 4.

Ingredients: Organic, local or seasonal
Red or regular quinoa (keen – wah) - 1 cup
Yellow onion – 1, medium sized, medium diced
Broccoli tops – ½ cup
Carrots – 2, small diced
Snow peas – ½ cup, de-stemmed, rough chopped
Rosemary powder – ½ tsp.
Thyme – ½ tsp.
"Cheesy Pleasy Sauce" - 4 Tbsps. (see page 79)
Sea salt – 1 tsp.
E.V. olive oil – 2 Tbsps.
Fresh cilantro leaves – 1 handful, rough chopped for garnish

Optional:
Garlic powder – 1 to 2 tsp.
Green onion – ¼ cup, rough chopped for garnish

Utensils: Chef's Knife, cutting board, prep bowls, large bowl to mix all together, bowl to soak quinoa, colander, measuring cup and spoons, flat spatula, serving platter, serving spoon, and stock bowl.

Directions:
- Soak the quinoa for a few minutes. Rinse and drain a few times in the colander.
- Rinse and prepare all the vegetables as above.
- In a saucepan, bring 2 cups water to a boil. Stir in the quinoa, a pinch of sea salt, turn heat down to low, and simmer until all the water evaporates (about 10 to 15 minutes).
- Remove the saucepan from heat and empty the contents into a large mixing bowl.

Stir-Fry:

- While the quinoa is cooking, warm a skillet on medium heat, add in the olive oil, chopped onions, spices, and stir-fry until slightly tender (about 3 to 4 minutes).
- Add in the broccoli, carrots, snow peas, and sauté lightly for 2 to 3 minutes.
- Stir in the "Cheesy Pleasy Sauce" and allow it to soften and become more creamy.
- Remove the skillet from heat.
- In a large mixing bowl, mix in the skillet contents with the finished quinoa.
- Taste and adjust seasonings.
- If you prefer more of the "Cheesy Pleasy" sauce, keep some extra warmed in a saucepan to add in at the end.
- Plate, garnish with a sprinkle of chopped green onion, and serve warm.

Note: Cooked red quinoa has a heartier, nuttier flavor and a chewier texture than the common golden variety.

Chickpea Spinach Curry

If you enjoy Indian cuisine, you'll love this rendition of Channa Saag. For a nice variation, try serving it over a bed of quinoa flavored with some cumin seeds and a squeeze of lime. It's a good way to increase the protein content and enhance the presentation. Curry powders, like the one used in this recipe, have many health-promoting properties. Its distinctive yellow-orange color comes from the herb turmeric. Turmeric contains a substance called curcumin. It supports healthy liver function, acts as a potent antioxidant and a powerful, natural anti-inflammatory substance in the body. Prep time: 40 to 45 minutes. Serves 4 to 6.

Ingredients: Organic, local or seasonal
Chickpeas – 2 cups, rinsed (cooked fresh or canned variety)
Yellow onion – 1, medium dice
Spinach leaves – 2, 6 oz. bags or 1lb bag frozen (thawed)
Garlic cloves – 4, rough chopped
Frozen green peas – ½ cup, thawed
Coconut milk – 1 cup, mixed with 1 cup water or vegetable stock
Curry masala powder – 3 Tbsps.
Thyme leaves – 1 tsp., (dried)
Sea salt – 2 tsp.
Extra virgin olive oil – 2 Tbsps. for the stir-fry, 2 Tbsps. for the sauce
Or substitute Earth Balance buttery spread – 2 Tbsps., for the sauce
Mesquite powder or brown rice flour – 3 Tbsps.
Lime – ½, fresh squeezed
Fennel seed powder – 1 tsp.
Cilantro – ¼ cup, rough chopped for garnish

Optional:
Cayenne powder – 1/8 tsp.
Green Curry paste – 1 tsp., ('Thai Kitchen' variety)

Utensils: Chef's knife, cutting board, prep bowls, large mixing bowl, large pot for soaking chick peas, large skillet or wok, measuring cup and measuring spoons, fine mesh strainer or colander, 3 quart saucepan or larger, colander, flat spatula or wooden spoon, and stock bowl.

Directions:
- Rinse and drain the chick peas.
- Prepare all vegetables as above and set in prep bowls prior to cooking.

Cooking:
- In a large saucepan on medium eat add in 2 to 3 Tbsps. olive oil.
- Stir-fry diced onions for 2 minutes, add in the sea salt, thyme, chopped garlic, fennel, and (optional) curry paste.
- With a spoon or spatula, clear the contents to one side of the pan and coat the empty part of pan with the oil (or butter).
- Using a whisk or spoon, quickly stir the mesquite in with the oil until it forms a paste. Stir in ½ cup vegetable stock or water to start the sauce.
- Pour in the coconut milk-stock mixture, 2 Tbsps. curry powder, stir well, and allow the sauce to thicken.
- Squeeze in the lime juice, stir in the chickpeas, and thawed green peas.
- If needed, adjust the amount and thickness of the sauce by adding in more coconut milk or vegetable stock or water.
- Taste and adjust the flavor with a few dashes of sea salt and/or curry powder.
- Keep warm on low heat.

Finishing:
- In a skillet or walk on medium heat, add ¼ cup vegetable stock or water and stir-fry the spinach until it reduces in size (about 3 to 4 minutes).
- Remove it from heat, drain the spinach well and mix it in with the finished ingredients in the large saucepan.
- Plate and serve atop of a bed of brown basmati rice or quinoa, and garnish with chopped cilantro.

Tip: For a spicier finish, add an additional teaspoon of curry paste to the stir–fry. Or, to help ease up on the spices, add an extra teaspoon or two of lime juice and/or a few ounces of coconut milk to adjust the spice level.

Holiday Loaf with Brown Sauce

This gourmet dish is an excellent entrée option for a holiday meal, special occasion or for entertaining guests. It provides significant sources of protein, fiber, folate, iron, molybdenum, manganese, magnesium, essential fats, and an appetizing golden brown sauce that might have you asking for seconds. Prep time – 1 hour. Serves 6 to 8.

Ingredients: Organic, local or seasonal
Quinoa – ¾ cup, soaked and rinsed
Navy beans – 1, 16oz. can, drained
Yellow onion – 1 medium size, rough chopped small
Fennel bulb – ½ cup, cored, rough chopped
Green onion – ½ cup, rough chopped
Garlic cloves – 2 or 3, minced
Sage – 2 Tbsps., powdered or rubbed
Rosemary – 1 tsp., chopped leaves or powdered
Thyme leaves – 1 tsp.
Flaxseed meal – ¼ cup
Sea salt – 2 tsp. (divided)
Extra virgin olive oil – 3 Tbsps..
Brown sauce (see page 81) – for garnish

Utensils: Chef's Knife, cutting board, 2 mixing bowls, bowl to soak quinoa, colander, masher or large fork, measuring cup and spoons, skillet, spatula or wooden spoon, rectangular 2" deep non-stick baking dish, serving platter, serving spatula, and stock bowl.

Directions:
- Preheat the oven to 350.
- Soak the quinoa for a few minutes. Rinse and drain in a colander a few times.
- Prepare the vegetables as above.
- Bring 1½ cups water to a boil, add a pinch of sea salt, stir in quinoa, turn the heat down to low, and cook until all the water is absorbed (about 10 to 15 minutes).
- Remove the quinoa from heat and let it cool in a large mixing bowl.

Stir-fry
- In a skillet on medium heat, add in the olive oil, onions, and stir-fry for 3 to 4 minutes.

- Add in the chopped fennel, garlic, sea salt, all other spices, and stir for 2 to 3 minutes.
- Remove the skillet from heat and set aside.

Mixing and Baking*:
- In another mixing bowl, mash the beans until soft and mostly smooth.
- Using a large spoon or spatula, fold in the quinoa, vegetable stir-fry contents, flax meal, and the green onions.
- Taste the mixture and adjust the seasonings if desired.
- Pack the contents about 2" high into a non-stick, rectangular baking dish, sprinkle sage over the top, cover with foil, and bake for 20 to 25 minutes.
- Remove foil and bake for an addition 20 to 25 minutes or until golden brown on top.
- Remove from the oven and let cool for a few minutes.
- Slice into 1" wide pieces with a metal spatula or paring knife and remove from the pan.
- To plate, ladle brown sauce over the top, garnish with a few sprinkles of chives, and serve.

*Baking option – For a more visual presentation, pack the mixture into individual, 1" h x 3" w non-stick baking molds or 6 oz. ramekins, and place them on a baking sheet to bake in the oven. Note that the cooking time will be shorter than the using the baking dish method so check periodically for desired results.

Holiday Quinoa

Paying tribute to the holiday theme, this recipe came about as a result of experimenting with quinoa and discovering many possible variations using this delightful food. It's a nice option to have for those that prefer having additional plant-based menu options around the holidays. Prep time 25 to 30 minutes. Serves 4 to 6.

Ingredients: Organic, local or seasonal
Quinoa (keen–wah) - 1 cup, soaked and rinsed, (regular or red variety)
Extra virgin olive oil – 2 Tbsps.
Yellow onion – 1, medium diced
Sea salt – 1 tsp.
Sage powder – 1 tsp.
Thyme – 1 tsp.
Cumin powder – 1 tsp.
Sun-dried tomato – ½ cup (whole-size), rough chopped
Garlic cloves – 4, rough chopped small
Frozen green peas – 1 cup, thawed

Optional:
Curley parsley – rough chopped for garnish

Utensils: Chef's Knife, cutting board, prep bowls, large mixing bowl, bowl to soak quinoa, colander, measuring cup and spoons, flat spatula, skillet, wire mesh strainer, saucepan, serving platter and spoon, and stock bowl.

Directions:
- Soak the quinoa for a few minutes. Rinse and drain a few times in the colander.
- In a saucepan, bring 2 cups water to a boil, add a pinch of sea salt, quinoa, and simmer on low heat until all water evaporates (about 15 to 20 minutes).
- While the quinoa is simmering, prepare the vegetables as above and set in prep bowls.
- When finished, remove the quinoa from the heat, fluff lightly with a fork, and let cool in large bowl.

Stir-fry:
- In a skillet on medium heat, add olive oil, onions, all spices, and stir for 3 to 4 minutes.

- Add in the sun-dried tomato, chopped garlic and stir for 2 to 3 minutes.
- Remove from heat and set aside.

Finishing:
- In the mixing bowl, fold in the green peas, skillet contents, and combine with the quinoa.
- Taste and adjust the seasonings if desired.
- Garnish with parsley and serve warm or chilled.

Tip: The finished quinoa should have a light, nutty flavor and a fluffy texture.

Add Your Own Recipe Ideas Here:

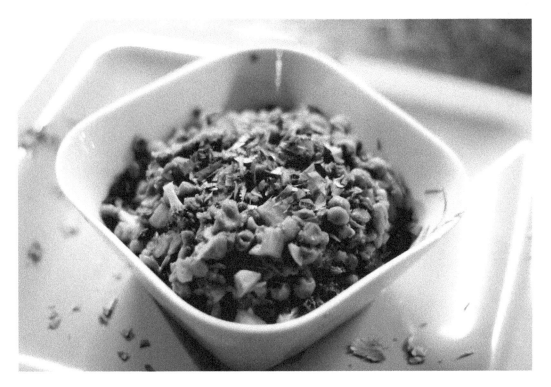

In No hurry Curry Lentils

In No Hurry Curry Lentils

Lentils are jam-packed with nearly 18 grams of protein per cup cooked and are excellent sources of folate, magnesium, phosphorus, potassium, and fiber to name a few. Although this is likely the most involved recipe in the book, the time and effort spent preparing it are absolutely worth the deliciousness at the end. It's also one of my favorite meals to serve for satisfying most, if not all, the tastes of the palate. Prep time: 1¼ hours. Serves 4 to 6.

Ingredients: Organic, local or seasonal
Green lentils* – 1 cup, soaked and rinsed
Dried apricots – 6, soaked and rough chopped
Vegetable stock or water – 2 cups divided (½ for stir-fry, ½ for curry sauce)
Yellow onion – 1, small sized, medium diced
Sea salt – 2 tsp.
Cumin powder – 1 tsp.
Curry masala powder – 3 Tbsps. (divided)
Fennel powder – 1 tsp.
Ginger root – 1" piece, minced
Garlic cloves – 6, rough chopped
Earth Balance buttery spread – 2 Tbsps.
Brown rice flour – 3 Tbsps. or mix with ½ mesquite powder
Coconut milk – 1¼ cups, dilute with ½ cup of vegetable stock or water
Lime juice – ½, fresh squeezed
Carrots – ½ cup, sliced into thin half moons
Broccoli tops – ¾ cup
Frozen peas – ½ cup, thawed

Optional:
Cilantro leaves – rough chopped for garnish
Green curry paste – (Thai kitchen) – 1 tsp., (add when stir-frying in skillet)
Sweet potato – 1 small, peeled, small diced, steamed or boiled

Utensils: Chef's knife, cutting board, prep bowls, large mixing bowl, small bowl for soaking, measuring cup and measuring spoons, citrus reamer or juicer, small whisk or spoon, colander, large saucepan, large skillet, peeler, flat spatula or wooden spoon, stock bowl.

*To save time, cook the lentils the night before and refrigerate them in a sealed container.

Directions:
- Soak the lentils in water for 5 to 10 minutes. Rinse and drain.
- Soak apricots in a bowl of warm water and set aside to soften.
- Rinse, drain and thaw the veggies as needed.
- Cut all vegetables as above, juice the lime, and set all in prep bowls before cooking.

Cooking:
- In a large saucepan, bring 2 cups water to a boil. Add in the lentils, 1 tsp. sea salt, turn down heat to low, simmer until all water evaporates (about 45 to 50 minutes), and the lentils are soft and chewy.
- While the lentils are simmering, warm a large skillet on medium heat. Add in the stock, diced onions, minced ginger, sea salt, cumin, 1 Tbsp. of curry powder, ground fennel, chopped garlic, and stir-fry for 2 to 3 minutes.

Pan curry sauce:
- Move the skillet contents to one-side of the pan. Melt in the earth balance butter, add the brown rice flour, and whisk quickly until brown and pasty.
- Whisk in a few ounces of vegetable stock, half the coconut milk, 2 Tbsps. curry powder, lime juice, and stir well.
- Bring the skillet to a simmer, stir and allow the sauce to thicken.
- As the sauce thickens, stir in the remaining coconut milk and additional stock to expand the amount of sauce.
- Mix in the remaining vegetables, apricots, stir well for 2 to 3 minutes, and remove the contents from the heat.

Finishing:
- In a large saucepan, mix the skillet contents in with the finished lentils and keep warm.
- Taste and adjust the flavor with additional curry powder or a few dashes of sea salt if desired.
- Serve warm, atop a bed of steamed brown basmati rice seasoned with a squeeze of lime juice, and a few dashes of cumin. Or, use cooked quinoa or millet in place of the rice.
- Garnish with chopped cilantro and serve warm.

Tip: For some extra heat, add 1 tsp. of green curry paste during the stir-fry step. Or, to help ease up on the spices, add in an extra tablespoon lime juice and/or a few ounces coconut milk.

Add Your Own Recipe Ideas Here:

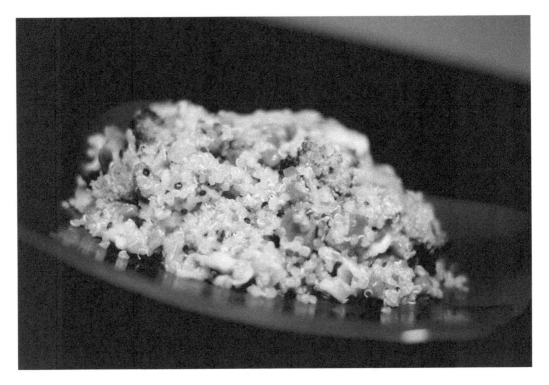

Magic Quinoa

Magic Quinoa

My first original recipe and an award winner, magic quinoa provides a simple yet enjoyable and cost effective choice for the weekly menu. I have prepared it for countless food demonstrations and it has always gone over well with the crowd. It's light and satisfying, has a pleasant savory flavor, provides the essential amino acids, essential fats, and ample amounts of fiber. Total prep time: 40 minutes. Serves 4 to 6.

Ingredients: Organic, local or seasonal
Quinoa – 1 cup, soaked and rinsed
Yellow onion – 1, medium diced
Green cabbage – ½ small head, cored and rough chopped small
Frozen peas – 1 cup, thawed
Carrots – 1, rough chopped small
Broccoli tops – ½ cup
Ginger root – 1" to 2" piece, minced
Garlic cloves – 3, minced
Rosemary powder – 1 tsp.
Thyme – 1 tsp.
Flax oil – 2 Tbsps. (Barlean's or Flora brand)
Sea salt – 2 tsp.

Optional:
Fennel bulb – ½ bulb (rough chop bulb part and add to stir-fry)
Lemon Zest - 1 tsp. (add into stir-fry)

Utensils: Chef's Knife, cutting board, prep bowls, large mixing bowl, bowl to soak the quinoa, colander, measuring cup and spoons, flat spatula, large skillet, large saucepan, serving platter, spoon, and stock bowl.

Directions:
- Soak the quinoa for a few minutes. Rinse and drain a few times in the colander.
- Rinse and prepare the vegetables as above.
- In a saucepan, bring 2 cups water to a boil, add in the quinoa, a pinch of sea salt, and simmer on low until all water has been absorbed (about 10 to 15 minutes). Remove from heat.
- Empty the contents into a mixing bowl, fluff lightly with a fork, and let cool.

Stir-Fry:
- In a skillet on medium heat, add olive oil, onions, and stir-fry for 2 to 3 minutes.
- Add in sea salt, thyme, minced ginger root, minced garlic, rosemary, cabbage, carrots, broccoli, and stir-fry for 3 to 4 minutes.
- Remove from heat and let cool.

Finishing:
- In the mixing bowl, stir the flax oil in with the quinoa.
- Add in thawed peas, skillet contents, and mix well.
- Taste and adjust the seasonings.
- Plate and garnish with chopped parsley, and serve warm.

Tip: For a different presentation idea, try serving the quinoa wrapped up in a warmed Ezekiel tortilla or a leaf of savoy cabbage.

Mama's Millet Chili

No matter what type of diet you follow, this recipe satisfies an appetite for a hearty meal, and it's a deliciously satisfying choice for chili lovers. One twelve ounce serving provides nearly half the adult daily protein requirement. It also contains notable amounts of folate, important minerals like magnesium, phosphorus, potassium and iron, great sources of complex carbohydrates, significant amounts of fabulous fiber, and takes about 40 minutes to prepare. Serves 6 to 8.

Ingredients: Organic, local or seasonal
Extra virgin olive oil – 2 Tbsps.
Sea salt – 2 tsp.
Sweet onion – 1, medium diced
Cumin powder – 2 to 3 tsp.
Chili powder - 2 to 3 Tbsps.
Lime – ½, juiced
Green or red pepper – 1, cored and seeded, rough chopped
Jalapeno pepper - 2, cored and seeded, rough chopped
Vegetable stock or water – 2 cups
Diced tomatoes – 2 x 15oz. cans (fire roasted if available)
Hulled millet – ¾ cup, rinsed
Red kidney beans* – 1, 16oz. organic canned variety
Northern beans* – 1, 16oz. organic canned variety
Black beans* – 1, 16oz. organic canned variety
Green onions – ¼ cup, rough chopped

*Any multiple-bean, organic canned variety will work. - 2 to 3, 16 oz. cans

Optional:
Cayenne powder – a few dashes
Corn kernels – ½ cup (fresh or frozen organic)

Utensils: Chef's knife, cutting board, measuring cup and spoons, colander, skillet, prep bowls, large soup pot, large slotted spoon, flat spatula, citrus reamer or juicer, and stock bowl.

Directions:
- Rinse the millet a few times and drain in a colander or wire mesh strainer.
- In a medium saucepan bring 3 cups water to a boil, add in a pinch of sea salt, the millet, turn the heat to low, and simmer. Cook the millet until all

the water evaporates (about 25 minutes), and immediately remove it from heat.
- Rinse and drain the beans in the colander.
- While the millet is coking, cut all the vegetables as above place in prep bowls.

Stir-Fry:
- In a large saucepan or soup pot on medium heat, add in the olive oil, onions, 1 tsp. sea salt, 1 tsp. cumin, 1 Tbsp. chili powder, the chopped vegetables, canned diced tomatoes, lime juice, and stir-fry for 3 to 4 minutes.
- Pour in the vegetable broth, the cooked millet and simmer on low heat.

Finishing:
- Stir in the beans and simmer on low heat for 5 to 10 minutes.
- Taste and adjust flavor with an additional Tbsp. or two of chili powder, 1 tsp. cumin, 1 tsp. of sea salt, and a few dashes of cayenne if desired.
- Plate, garnish with a few sprinkles of green onions, "Crunchies" or wrap some up in a soft Ezekiel tortilla, and enjoy.

Mexican Quinoa

The more you experiment with this terrific little seed-grain the more variations you will discover. That's exactly what happened when I came up with this recipe. Because of its wonderful colors, textures and tastes, this dish has always been a great choice to feature in my food demonstrations. Like the other recipes using quinoa in this book, you'll enjoy the taste, nutrition, and the option of having another way to prepare this versatile food. Prep time: 30 to 35 minutes. Serves 4 to 6.

Ingredients: Organic, local or seasonal
Quinoa (Keen–wah) - 1 cup, soaked and rinsed, (regular or red variety)
Yellow onion, 1 – medium diced
Red peppers – 1, rough chopped
Jalapeño pepper – 1, minced
Chile powder – 2 Tbsps.
Cumin powder – 1 tsp.
Extra virgin olive oil – 4 Tbsps.
Black beans – ¾ cup, organic, canned variety, rinsed
Corn – ½ cup, organic, fresh or frozen
Lime juice – 2 Tbsps., fresh squeezed
Sea salt – 1 tsp.

Optional:
Savoy cabbage* – 1 small head, leaves separated
Lime zest - 1 Tbsp., added to stir-fry
Cayenne pepper – one or two dashes
Jicama – small dice, for garnish

Utensils: Chef's Knife, cutting board, large mixing bowl, bowl to soak quinoa, mesh strainer or colander, measuring cup and spoons, flat spatula, skillet, wire mesh strainer, saucepan, serving platter and spoon, and stock bowl.

Directions:
- Soak the quinoa for about 5 minutes. Rinse and drain a few times in a mesh strainer.
- In a saucepan, bring 2 cups water to a boil, add a pinch of sea salt, quinoa, and simmer on low heat until the water is absorbed (about 10 to 15 minutes).
- While the quinoa simmers, rinse and prepare the vegetables as above.
- Remove the quinoa from heat and let cool in a large mixing bowl.

Stir-fry:
- In a skillet on medium heat, add the olive oil, the onions, and stir-fry for 3 to 4 minutes.
- Add in the sea salt, chili powder, cumin, jalapeños, red peppers, lime juice, and stir-fry until slightly tender (about 3 to 4 minutes). Remove from heat and let cool.

Finishing:
- In a large bowl, mix together the beans, corn, and skillet contents with the finished quinoa.
- Taste and adjust seasonings if desired.
- Empty contents into a large saucepan and keep warm prior to serving.
- Plate, garnish as desired, and serve warm or chilled.

*Serving tip: For a nice serving variation, plate the finished quinoa wrapped inside a leaf of savoy cabbage. Garnish with some small diced jicama and lime zest. It's a simple way to add visual appeal, elegance, flavor, and better nutrition to your meal.

Add Your Own Recipe Ideas Here:

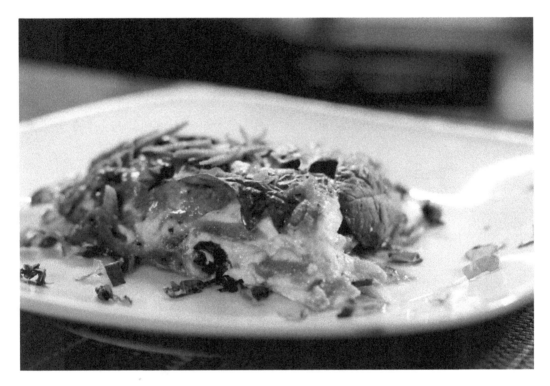

Mostly Raw Lasagna

Mostly Raw Lasagna

This more natural approach to traditional lasagna is completely dairy and gluten-free. Inspired by my love of Italian foods, this delicious dish is full of flavor, a smooth, creamy texture, and great nutrition. While the nut based cheese it contains offer good sources of protein and beneficial essential fatty-acids, the zucchini and yellow squash provide quality amounts of vitamin A, folate, potassium, fiber, and are naturally low in carbohydrates. For those who would prefer to enjoy lasagna without indulging in additional carbohydrates, this recipe offers a yummy yet practical substitute. Prep time: 45 minutes. Serves 4 to 6.

Ingredients: Organic, local or seasonal
Red sauce – 1, 16 oz. (or larger) jar, tomato basil variety
"Almost Ricotta Cheeze" sauce – 1½ cups (see page 75)
Zucchini – 1, sliced very thin, long ways
Yellow squash – 1, sliced very thin, long ways
Carrots – 1, shredded
Spinach leaves – 5 oz. bag
Extra virgin olive oil or flax oil
Fresh basil leaves – 1 small handful, chopped small

Optional:
Oregano – sprinkled for garnish

Utensils: Chef's knife, cutting board, prep bowls, large mixing bowl, measuring cup and measuring spoons, peeler or mandolin slicer, 9 X 9 deep dish pan, colander, pastry brush, serving spatula, large spoon, and stock bowl.

Directions:
- The night before, prepare the "Almost Ricotta Cheeze", and keep refrigerated.

Tip: Before preparing this recipe, leave the sauce and cheeze out for 10 to 15 minutes to bring them to room temperature. This helps to spread them more easily.

- Rinse and prepare vegetables as above.

Preparing squash noodles:
- On a cutting board, cut off the ends of the squash and discard.
- Using a peeler or mandolin, slice the squash into very thin strips long ways (as to resemble a thin noodle). Set the slices in a large bowl or on a plate. You may discard the outer skins if desired.

Making the Lasagna:

- Before layering in the deep dish, coat the bottom of it with a thin layer of red sauce.
- Layer in the deep serving dish as follows:
- Place a layer of zucchini noodles (vertically) and overlap each of the noodles.
- Place the next layer of yellow squash (horizontally) over the zucchini overlapping each of the noodles.
- Gently spread on a layer of the cheeze with a pastry brush or large spoon.
- Spoon in a layer of the red sauce.
- Add on a thin layer of spinach leaves.
- Sprinkle on a thin layer of shredded carrots.
- Repeat as above one more time, and garnish with sprinkles of fresh basil, and oregano leaves as desired.

Finishing:

- Set the pan in a food dehydrator at 115 - 120 degrees and warm for 15 minutes before serving. Or, if a dehydrator is not available, warm it on the lowest temperature setting in a conventional oven for about 10 minutes prior to serving.

Serving:

Using a serving spatula, slice it into equal-sized squares, plate, and garnish with a few sprinkles of oregano, chopped fresh basil leaves, and serve.

My Thai Stir-fry

After finishing this recipe, you might feel like you went out to one of your favorite Thai restaurants for dinner. Although this sumptuous meal takes some extra time to prepare, you'll know after the first bite it was well worth the effort. In addition to the feeling of accomplishment, you'll appreciate the fact that this dish contains a significant amount of plant-based protein, monounsaturated fats, fiber, and bursts of flavor in every bite. Prep time: 35 to 40 minutes. Serves 6 to 8.

Ingredients: Organic, local or seasonal

Pad Thai noodles or zucchini noodles* – 8 oz. pkg. (international foods aisle)
Edamame beans (shelled soybeans) – 1½ cups, thawed (frozen foods aisle)
Yellow onion – 1, cored and julienne (thin, stick-like slices)
Fresh bean sprouts – 1 cup, (located in the fresh produce area)
Garlic cloves – 2, minced
Carrots – ½ cup, rough chopped
Ginger root – 1" piece, minced
Broccoli – 1 medium-sized crown, tops only – ¾ cup
Sesame oil – 3 Tbsps. for the stir-fry, ¼ cup for sauce
Wheat-free tamari – ¾ cup (international foods aisle)
Rice vinegar – ¼ cup (international foods aisle)
Sesame seeds – white or black variety – 2 Tbsps. for garnish
Chili paste – 1 tsp., from 'Thai Kitchen' (international foods aisle)

Optional:

Organic extra-firm (sprouted) tofu 1 lb. pkg. - ½ pkg., drained, medium diced
*Zucchini – 2 large sized, sliced into noodles with julienne peeler

Utensils: Chef's knife, cutting board, colander, prep bowls, flat spatula or wooden spoon, large mixing bowl, large skillet or Wok, measuring spoons, measuring cups, colander, peeler, and stock bowl.

Directions:
- Thaw and rinse all veggies as needed.
- Rinse and cut the vegetables as above and place in prep bowls.

Cooking:
- In a large saucepan, bring 6 cups of water to a boil.
- Add in the noodles, a pinch of sea salt, and simmer on low heat.
  *(If using the zucchini noodles instead of rice noodles, steam them in the water until soft and slightly chewy: 5 to 6 minutes).

- Cook until the texture is soft and slightly chewy (about 5 to 6 minutes).
- Drain and set aside in a large mixing bowl.

Making the pad sauce:
- In a mixing bowl or large measuring cup, whisk together the rice vinegar, tamari, ginger, garlic, honey, and lastly, whisk in the sesame oil.

In a skillet or wok:
- In a large skillet or wok on medium heat, add in half of the pad sauce mixture, and stir in the chili paste.
- Add in any of the optional ingredients, onions, carrots, broccoli, edamame beans, bean sprouts, and stir for about 3 to 4 minutes.
- Add in the cooked noodles, the remaining pad sauce, and stir until well combined.
- Plate, sprinkle on the sesame seeds for garnish, and serve warm.

Add Your Own Recipe Ideas Here:

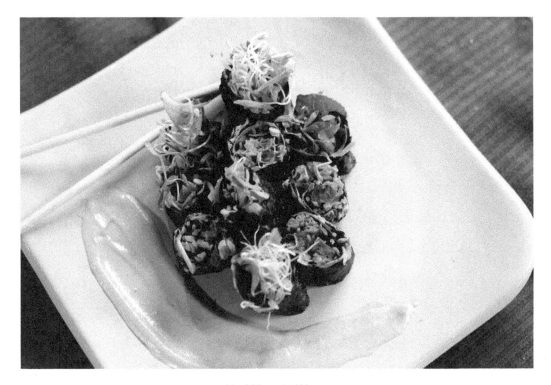

Nori Veggie Wrap

Nori Veggie Wrap

Nori is a sea vegetable that is most commonly used in Japanese cuisine to prepare sushi. It's the dark green looking sheets to which the sushi rice is applied and has a salty, sea like taste because it comes from the ocean. It also happens to be full of health sustaining nutrition and is a significant source of iodine, a good source of vitamin E, vitamin K, thiamin, pantothenic acid, vitamin A, vitamin C, riboflavin, niacin, vitamin B6, folate, iron, calcium, phosphorus, zinc, potassium, copper, manganese, and protein. All things aside, this delicious wrap is fun and easy to prepare, and makes a beautiful presentation for any occasion. Prep time: 20 to 25 minutes. Serves 4 to 6.

Ingredients: Organic, local or seasonal
Nori Sheets – 1 pkg., (from Asian food store or health food store)
Carrots - 1, shredded
Sprouts – ½ cup, broccoli, clover or sunflower (fresh produce area)
"Cheesy Pleasy Sauce" - spread as needed (see page 79)
Tomato – 1, roma or vine ripe, cored, seeded, and rough chopped
Bibb lettuce, spinach, or mixed salad greens – small bag
Raw honey – spread as needed to close the wrap
Wheat-free tamari – drizzle on top for garnish

Optional:
Avocado – pitted, scooped, and thinly sliced
Savoy cabbage – 1 head, leaves separated (substitute for the nori if desired)

Utensils: Chef's knife, cutting board, serrated knife, box shredder, prep bowls, colander, rubber spatula and pastry brush, sushi rolling mat, serrated knife, and stock bowl.

Directions:
- In a large colander, rinse and drain the sprouts, and lightly pat them dry with a towel.
- Prepare the vegetables as above and place in prep bowls.
- On top of a cutting board or a sushi rolling mat, layout one nori sheet, spread on a thin layer of "Cheesy Pleasy Sauce" with a spatula and leave about ¼" at the top end empty.
- Make a thin layer of each of the following: spinach or mixed greens, tomatoes, shredded carrots, sprouts, and cover with any optional ingredients.

- Using a pastry brush, apply a thin layer of raw honey to the top end of the nori sheet.
- Using both hands, gently roll the nori sheet carefully toward the top, and secure the top as you finish.
- Using a serrated knife, cut the roll in half four times to make eight equal-sized pieces.
- Plate with the open side up, garnish with a drizzle of tamari sauce, "Cheesy Pleasy Sauce", and serve with your favorite soup.

Tip: For a nice decorative variation, try using a piece of savoy cabbage instead of the nori.

You can also tie off the wrap with a thin strip of nori or just fold it by hand and enjoy. It adds a nice visual appeal, a nice crunch and extra good nutrition.

Polenta Lasagna

Polenta has been a popular choice in fine dining restaurants for years. This recipe is another variation on this classic Italian dish and you won't miss the pasta noodles. It's a great meal for entertaining guests or for that special someone in your life. This dish was also a runner up in an annual recipe competition sponsored by Food and Wine magazine. If you prefer not to use goat cheese, feel free to substitute it with "Almost Ricotta Cheeze". Prep Time: 50 to 55 minutes. Serves 4 to 6 adults.

Ingredients: Organic, local or seasonal
Polenta – 1, 18 oz. loaf*, ¼" wide slices (makes 18 to 20 pieces per loaf)
Yellow onion – 1, cored, julienne (thin, stick-like slices), caramelized
Carrots – 1 large, shredded
Spinach leaves – 3 to 4 cups (5 oz. bag fresh spinach leaves)
Fresh local goat cheese - 4 oz. pkg. or "Almost Ricotta Cheeze" (see page 75)
Red sauce – 26 oz. jar, tomato basil variety
Garlic cloves – 4, rough chopped
Sea salt – 1 tsp.
White pepper – 1 dash
Extra virgin olive oil – 3 Tbsps.
Fresh basil leaves – a handful, shredded for garnish

Optional:
Shredded mozzarella – for garnish, (Daiya – non-dairy brand)

Utensils: Chef's knife, cutting board, prep bowls, large mixing bowl, large skillet or wok, measuring cup and measuring spoons, 9"x 9" square deep baking dish, colander, flat serving spatula, wooden spoon, box shredder, aluminum foil, and stock bowl.

Directions:
- Pre-heat the oven to 350.
- Prepare the polenta, vegetables as above, and set them in prep bowls prior to cooking.

On the stovetop:
- In a skillet on medium heat, add in the olive oil, sliced onions, sea salt, a dash of pepper, and let them caramelize (about 12 to 15 minutes).
- Stir the onions occasionally, cook until very soft, and brown.
- Remove the skillet from heat and let the onions cool for a few minutes.
- Rough chop the onions and put them into a mixing bowl.

- Using the same skillet on medium heat, add 2 Tbsps. olive oil, garlic, carrots, thawed or fresh spinach and stir fry for 3 to 4 minutes or until the spinach reduces.
- Remove the skillet from heat and drain the mixture of extra moisture in a colander.
- Combine the spinach contents with the caramelized onions.

Layering in the baking dish:
- Coat the bottom of the baking dish with a thin layer of red sauce.
- Layer in the following manner:
  Polenta*, red sauce, sautéed vegetable mixture, goat cheese**, (mozzarella)
  Repeat once.

Baking and serving:
- Cover the dish with aluminum foil, place in oven, and set baking time alarm for 20 minutes.
- After 20 minutes, remove the foil and bake for an additional 10 to 15 minutes.
- Remove it from the oven and let cool for a few minutes.
- Using a metal serving spatula or utility knife, cut the lasagna into even squares, plate, garnish with sprinkles of shredded fresh basil leaves, and serve.

*One polenta loaf will supply enough for two full layers. It's best to use an organic, non-GMO variety from the store. Or, if you are a more experienced chef, make your own polenta at home.

**To apply the goat cheese layer, use a spreading knife or teaspoon to cut small slices and apply them by hand. Fresh goat cheese is easier to apply when chilled.

Simple Tofu Stir-Fry

Simple, delicious and timely to prepare, this is an ideal recipe for any day of the week. Organic, non-GMO tofu is an excellent source of protein, calcium, magnesium, iron, potassium, selenium, and phosphorus, etc., and adds color and texture to different recipes. Prep time: 15 minutes. Serves 4 to 6.

Ingredients: Organic, local or seasonal
Pre-cut vegetable mix – 1 lb. pkg., from produce area or frozen
Extra-firm tofu – 8 oz. pkg., (sprouted or regular), drained, medium diced
Extra virgin olive oil – 3 Tbsps. or vegetable broth – ½ cup as needed
Thyme leaves – 1 tsp., dried or fresh
Garlic powder – ½ tsp.
Sea Salt - 1 tsp.
Cayenne Pepper - 1 pinch

Optional:
Lemon zest – 1 Tbsp.
Red miso paste – 1 Tbsp., added to the stir-fry to deepen the flavor
Parsley – rough chopped for garnish

Utensils: Chef's knife, cutting board, prep bowls, large skillet, wooden spoon, colander, 2 salad plates, measuring spoons, serving platter, stock bowl, and a healthy appetite.

Directions:
- Over the sink, gently press the tofu between two salad plates to remove any excess water.
- Dice the tofu as above.

Stir-Fry:
- In a skillet on medium heat, add olive oil or broth, tofu, stir occasionally for 8 to 10 minutes, or until light brown on two sides. Remove and set aside in a prep bowl.

Tip: As the tofu tends to stick very easily, use a non-toxic, reliable, non-stick pan, and keep enough olive oil or broth to keep the pan moist.
- In the same skillet, add in the mixed vegetables, all spices, miso, and stir-fry for 3 to 4 minutes. If necessary, add an extra Tbsp. olive oil or a few Tbsp. of vegetable broth to coat bottom of the skillet.

- Mix the cooked tofu cubes back in with the skillet contents, and stir for 1 to 2 minutes.
- Taste, adjust seasonings, and remove from heat.
- Plate and garnish as desired and serve warm.

Soba Florentine

This recipe offers a flavorsome alternative to the traditional pasta meal theme. If you really enjoy pasta but have wheat allergies or sensitivities, this dish is worth trying. Buckwheat is really more like a fruit seed and is related to rhubarb and sorrel. For many with wheat allergies, it's okay to eat because it's naturally gluten-free. It also contains good amounts of protein, fiber, folate, magnesium, and potassium, etc. Prep time: 30 to 35 minutes. Serves 6 to 8.

Ingredients: Organic, local or seasonal
Buckwheat soba noodles – 8 oz. pkg. (international foods aisle)
Yellow onion – 1, medium diced
Carrots – 1 cup, sliced into half-moons ¼ "wide
Snow peas – ½ cup, end stems snapped off, sliced into quarters
Spinach leaves – 2 (5 oz. pkgs. or 1 large size pkg.)
Sea salt – 1 tsp.
Thyme – 1 to 2 tsps.
Fresh basil leaves – 1 Tbsp., chopped small for garnish
Extra virgin olive oil - 2 Tbsps. (for stir-fry) or vegetable broth – ½ cup
Red sauce – 1, 28 oz. jar, organic or local variety

Sauce* Ingredients
Whole or diced roma tomatoes – 1 can, 28 oz.
Extra virgin olive oil – ¼ cup
Yellow onion – 1, small diced
Garlic – 2 large cloves (or 3 small), minced
Oregano Leaves – dried, 1 to 2 tsp.
Basil Leaves – fresh or dried, 1 to 2 tsp.
Sea Salt – 1 tsp.
Lemon juice – 2 tsp.
Water – 1 cup

Optional:
Lima Beans - ½ cup (fresh or frozen)
Broccoli tops – ½ cup (fresh or frozen)

Utensils: Chef's knife, cutting board, colander, prep bowls, flat spatula or wooden spoon, large mixing bowl, large skillet or Wok, medium sauce pan, large saucepan, measuring spoons, peeler, ladle, and stock bowl.

Directions:
- Rinse and prepare all vegetables as above, and set aside in prep bowls.
- In a saucepan on low heat, simmer the red sauce until ready to serve.

Cooking the soba:
- In large sauce pan, boil 6 cups of water, break noodles in half, add them in with a pinch of sea salt and turn the heat down to low.
- Cook until texture is soft and slightly chewy (about 5 to 6 minutes).
- Rinse the soba with cold water, drain, and put it in a large mixing bowl.

Stir-fry:
- In a skillet on medium heat, add in the olive oil, diced onion, sea salt, thyme, and stir-fry for 3 minutes.
- Add in carrots, snow peas, and stir fry for 3 to 4 minutes.
- Mix the skillet contents into mixing bowl with the soba noodles.
- In the same skillet, add olive oil or stock and stir-fry the spinach until it has reduced in size (about 2 to 3 minutes). Remove from heat.
- Drain the cooked spinach in a colander.
- Mix in the spinach with the cooked vegetables, and soba.

Serving:
- Plate, ladle the sauce over top, add garnish, and serve warm.

*Sauce Directions:
- In a medium saucepan on medium heat, add in 3 Tbsps. olive oil, chopped onions, garlic cloves, oregano, basil, sea salt, and sauté for 3 to 4 minutes.
- Add in the contents of canned tomatoes, water, and simmer on low heat.
- Taste and adjust seasonings.

Tip: For a smoother texture, pour the sauce contents into a food processor or blender and mix until desired texture is reached. For a lighter flavor on the taste buds, add the juice from half of a fresh lemon.

Add Your Own Recipe Ideas Here:

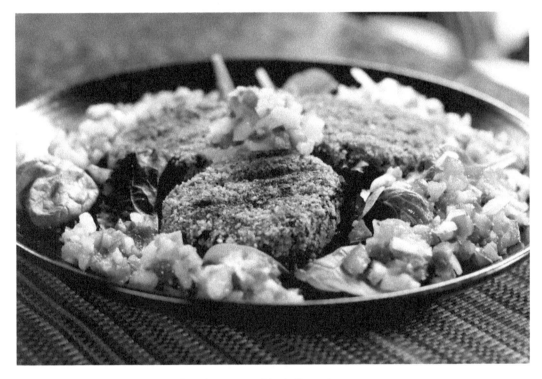

Southwestern Black Bean burger

Southwestern Black Bean Burger

If you are looking for a good quality protein option, this recipe offers ample amounts. Black beans are also significant sources of folate, magnesium, iron and fiber. It's one of my favorite recipes to make for clients and satisfies some of the most skeptical black bean burger aficionados. Prep time: 40 - 45 minutes. Makes 12 to 14 patties.

Ingredients: Organic, local or seasonal
Black beans – 2, 16 oz. cans, rinsed, and drained
Yellow onion – 1, rough chopped
Red pepper – 1, cored and seeded, rough chopped
Jalapeno pepper – 1 or 2, small, cored, seeded, and rough chopped
Bread crumbs – 1½ cups (1 cup for burger mix, ½ cup to finish) – 5 to 6 toasted slices (Ezekiel 4:9 sprouted bread or a package of gluten-free bread crumbs)
Flaxseed meal – ¼ cup
Chili powder - 2 Tbsps.
Cumin powder – 2 tsp.
Cayenne pepper – a few dashes (add to the bread crumbs or burger mix)
Fresh squeezed lime juice – 1 lime
Extra virgin olive oil – 2 Tbsps.
Sea salt – 2 tsp.

Optional:
Fennel bulb – ½ rough chopped (add it to the stir-fry step)
"Chunky Mango Salsa" (see page 31) – for garnish as desired

Utensils: Chef's knife, cutting board, large skillet, measuring cup and spoons, large mixing bowl, food processor or blender, citrus reamer or juicer, prep bowls, large fork or masher, flat spatula, and stock bowl.

Directions:
- Pre-heat the oven to 350.
- Rinse and drain the beans and place them into a large mixing bowl.
- Cut all the vegetables as above place in prep bowls.
- Put all the vegetables into food processor and pulse until chopped small.

Bread Crumbs:
- Toast the bread slices until golden brown and grind in food processor into very fine crumbs.

- Mix in 1 Tbsp. chili powder, 1 tsp. sea salt, 1 tsp. cumin, a few dashes of cayenne (if desired) into the bread crumbs, and set aside.
- Set ½ cup of bread crumbs aside for garnishing the patties prior to cooking.

Stir-Fry:
- In a skillet on medium heat, add 3 Tbsps. olive oil, onions, 1 tsp. sea salt, 1 tsp. cumin,
  1 Tbsp. chili powder, all chopped vegetables, lime juice, and stir fry for 3 to 4 minutes.
- Remove the skillet from heat and let cool.

Burger Mix:
- In mixing bowl, mash the black beans with a fork or masher until mostly smooth.
- Mix in all the skillet contents.
- Using your hands or flat spatula, fold in the bread crumbs, flax meal, and combine well.
- Taste the mixture, adjust seasonings and add in a dash or two of cayenne powder if desired.

Making the Patties:
- Form tightly into ½" thick, palm sized patties, and garnish with a thin layer of bread crumbs.

Tip: Before applying bread crumbs, brush a little water on the burgers with a pastry brush or your hands so the bread crumbs stick more easily.

Baking*:
- Place the patties on a non-stick baking sheet and bake at 350 until golden brown and crispy on top (about 25 to 30 minutes).

Serving:
- Plate atop a bed of mixed greens and top the burger with salsa or a spread of "Cheesy Pleasy Sauce". Serve with or without whole grain buns, and top with a slice of tomato or caramelized sweet onions if desired.

*To save cooking time and add a crispy finish, the patties may be cooked on an outdoor grill or Foreman style grill for 5 to 6 minutes.

Add Your Own Recipe Ideas Here:

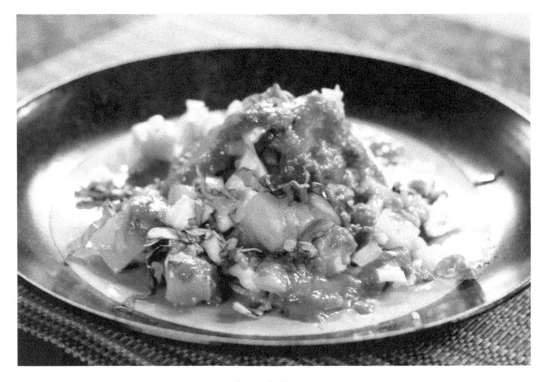

Squash Party

Squash Party

A squash lover's paradise! Spaghetti squash is an ideal substitute for pasta and great for those interested in foods lower in carbohydrates. If you have never tried spaghetti squash, you're in for a pleasant surprise. As its name suggests, it's remarkably similar in texture to pasta and yet it has its own unique and enjoyable flavor. This sumptuous dish is full of vitamin A, and a good source of vitamin C, folate, trace minerals, fiber, phytochemicals like lycopene, and immune system supporting herbs. Prep time: 55 to 60 minutes.
Serves 4 to 6.

Ingredients: Organic, local or seasonal
Spaghetti squash – 1, approx. 2 to 3 lbs
Butternut squash – 2 cups, small diced (pre-cut pkg. from produce if available)
Sea salt – 1 tsp.
Yellow squash – 1, medium sized, cut into ¼" wide half moons
Zucchini – 1, medium sized, cut into ¼" wide half moons
Garlic cloves – 4, rough chopped
Fennel bulb – ½ bulb part, cored, and rough chopped small
Fresh basil leaves – rough copped for garnish
Extra virgin olive oil – 4 Tbsps.
Tomato basil sauce - 26 oz. jar, organic or locally made sauce

Utensils: Chef's knife, paring knife, cutting board, colander, skillet, wooden spoon or flat spatula, large sauce pan, large mixing bowl, measuring cup, measuring spoons, large fork, large Pyrex or ceramic deep dish pan, and stock bowl.

Directions:
- Preheat the oven to 375.
- Rinse all produce and drain.
- Cut the spaghetti squash in half, scoop out, and compost the seeds.
- Fill a large baking sheet or deep dish pan with about ¼" water, place squash face down in the dish, and bake at 375 for about 40 minutes.
- While squash is baking, cut all other vegetables as above.
- To test the doneness of the squash, pierce it gently with a fork.

Stir-fry:
- In a skillet on medium heat, add olive oil, stir-in the onions, butternut squash cubes for 8 to 10 minutes.
- Add in 1 tsp. of sea salt and rosemary. The finished squash should be soft and tender.

- Mix in the chopped fennel, chopped garlic, zucchini, yellow squash, and stir fry for 2 to 3 minutes. Remove the pan from heat and let cool.

Finishing:
- Using a fork, gently scoop out spaghetti squash, and put contents into a large mixing bowl.
- Combine the stir fried vegetables with the spaghetti squash in the mixing bowl, and mix well.
- Plate, ladle on the tomato sauce, and garnish with fresh basil.

Serving tip: For a nice serving variation, keep the spaghetti squash separate from the other mixed squash at the end, and layer on the plate in the following manner:

Spaghetti squash
Ladle of tomato sauce
Mixed squash
Basil garnish

Add Your Own Recipe Ideas Here:

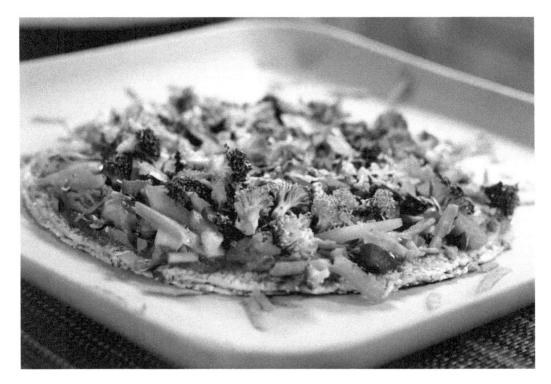

Veggie Pizza Quesadilla

Veggie Pizza Quesadilla

Although there's some extra prep needed to finish it, the time spent will be well worth it; especially if you are sensitive to processed wheat and dairy. If time is an issue, you can always follow the shortcuts that are indicated below*. To have some more fun making this recipe you can enlist a friend, partner or kids to help. More importantly, this savory dish provides an easy way to enjoy great flavors and the nutritional benefits of many vegetables in one meal. Total est. prep time: 60 minutes. Serves 2 to 4.

Ingredients: Organic, local or seasonal
Ezekiel tortillas or gluten-free variety – 1 pkg. (large size, 6 per pkg.)
(From frozen foods section at market or health food store)
Tomato basil sauce – 1, 16 oz. jar

Vegetable Toppings: (*Choose a pre-cut package from produce area)
Yellow onion – ½, small diced
Peppers – 1 of each, orange, yellow, red – sliced into ½" long, thin strips
Broccoli tops – ½ cup, crowns broken into small pieces
Carrots – ½ cup, shredded
Fresh cilantro leaves or fresh basil leaves – ¼ cup de-stemmed and rough chopped

Cheeze Ingredients: (*Prepare this recipe the night before)
Raw cashews – ¾ cup
Raw Brazil nuts or macadamia nuts – ¼ cup
Nutritional yeast – 1 Tbsp.
Garlic powder – ½ tsp.
Sea salt – ½ tsp. (optional)
Oregano – ½ tsp.
Cayenne pepper – (optional - 1 pinch)
Onion powder – ½ tsp.
Yellow miso paste – 2 Tbsps.
Lemon juice – 3 to 4 Tbsps.

Utensils: Chef's knife, cutting board, prep bowls, food processor or high speed blender, colander, measuring cup and spoons, flat spatula, pastry brush, pizza cutter, and stock bowl.

Directions:
- Rinse all vegetables, prepare them as above, and place in prep bowls.

Cheeze:
- In blender or food processor, mix all nuts into a fine powder.
- Add in the spices, nutritional yeast, and mix well.
- Mix in the lemon juice, miso paste, and blend until a smooth, spreadable texture is reached.
- Taste and adjust seasonings and thickness if desired.

Tip: The finished cheeze should be paste-like, smooth, and spreadable. If it comes out too thick, mix in an additional 1 or 2 tsp. lemon juice at the end.

Finishing the pizza:
- With a rubber spatula, spread one side of a tortilla with a layer of the cheeze and firmly press a second tortilla on top of it. They should stick together easily.
- Brush a light coating of olive oil on top of the tortilla and sprinkle on a few dashes of sea salt.
- Using a large spoon, cover the top with a thin layer of red sauce and leave a ½" area around the edge of the tortilla plain.
- To finish, add a thin layer of each vegetable in the following order:
- Onions, shredded carrots, peppers, broccoli, cilantro or chopped fresh basil leaves, extra pieces of cheese, and a few dashes of oregano.

Serving:
- Serve chilled or try it warm by baking it lightly in the oven for 10 to 12 minutes at 275.
- Using a pizza cutter or chef's knife, slice it into eight equal triangles and serve.

Serving variation
- Cut the pizza into 4 equal sections.
- Carefully fold each piece in half.
- Place them on a baking sheet and warm it in the oven on the lowest temperature setting for about 10 to 15 minutes or until crispy on top.
- Serve in the traditional folded style and garnish with fresh cilantro or basil.

Variation:

Greek style: Follow the same directions as above and substitute the following vegetables:

Kalamata olives, ½ cup, pitted, drained, and rough chopped small

Artichoke hearts – organic canned variety – 2 hearts, rough chopped

Zucchini – 1 small sized, small diced

Yellow squash – 1 small sized, small diced

Sun-dried tomato – ¼ cup (whole size), pre-softened in warm water, rough chopped small

Fresh basil leaves – ¼ cup, fresh, rough chopped

Vivacious Veggie Bean Quinoa Patties

For the veggie burger lovers out there, you'll enjoy the zesty flavor of this recipe. In addition to the quality protein and fiber it contains, topping it with "Cheesy Pleasy Sauce" will enhance flavor, and add more eye-catching color to the finished dish. If you like a little more spice in your life, add in an extra chipotle or two. Prep time: 45 to 50 minutes. Makes 8 to 10 palm-sized patties.

Ingredients: Organic, local or seasonal
Quinoa – ¾ cup, soaked, rinsed, and drained
Vegetable stock or water – 1½ cups
White navy beans – 1, 15oz. can
Yellow onion – 1, rough chopped
Carrots – 1 large, shredded
Chipotle peppers in adobo sauce (7oz. can from market) – ¼ cup of the sauce, and 2 peppers minced
Garlic cloves – 3 to 4 cloves, rough chopped
Green onions – ½ cup, rough chopped
E.V. olive oil – 2 Tbsps.
Bread crumbs – 1 cup, divided (Ezekiel 4:9 sprouted bread), 4 toasted slices
Ground flaxseed – ¼ cup
Onion powder – 1 tsp.
Garlic powder – 1 tsp.
Sea salt – 1 tsp.

Optional:
"Cheesy Pleasy Sauce"– for garnish as desired
Cayenne powder – 2 pinches
Yellow onions – ½, caramelized

Utensils: Chef's knife, cutting board, medium saucepan, large skillet, measuring cup and spoons, large mixing bowl, prep bowls, small food processor or blender, large fork or masher, spatula, pair of food service gloves, and stock bowl.

Directions:
- Soak the quinoa for 5 minutes. Rinse and drain a few times.
- Rinse the vegetables and the beans.

- In a saucepan, bring 2 cups of the water or vegetable stock to a boil, add 1 teaspoon of sea salt, quinoa, and simmer for about 15 minutes or until all water is absorbed. When done remove from heat and place the contents into a mixing bowl.
- While the quinoa is cooking, prepare the vegetables as above and place beans in the large mixing bowl.

Making the herbed bread crumbs:
- Toast the bread slices until golden brown.
- In the food processor or blender, grind the bread slices into fine crumbs, and mix in the following seasonings: 1 tsp. of sea salt, 1/8 tsp. white or black pepper, 1 tsp. thyme leaves, 1 tsp. onion powder, 1 tsp. garlic powder, and optional cayenne powder.
- Empty the contents into a prep bowl.

Stir-Fry:
- Preheat the oven to 350.
- In a skillet on medium heat, add in the olive oil, all spices, chipotle sauce, the chopped vegetables, and stir-fry for 2 to 3 minutes. Remove the skillet from heat and set aside.
- Spoon the skillet contents into the food processor and pulse a few times until small.

Making the patties:
- In a large mixing bowl, mash the beans with fork or masher until mostly smooth, and mix in half the herbed bread crumbs by hand.
- Add the stir-fry chopped vegetables to the bean mixture, remaining bread crumbs, and mix well by hand.
- Taste the mixture and, if necessary, adjust seasonings.
- Wearing food services gloves, tightly pack into ½" thick, palm sized patties. There should be enough for approximately 8 to 10 patties.

Baking* the patties:
- Bake the patties at 350 on a non-stick, foil-lined baking sheet until golden brown, and crispy on top (about 30 to 35 minutes). Check periodically for doneness.

Serving:
- Serve on a bed of mixed greens topped with salsa or on Ezekiel 4:9 buns with lettuce and tomato and a side of "Baked Sweets" (page 113).
- Garnish with some "Cheesy Pleasy Sauce" (page 79) and a pinch or 2 of cayenne powder.

*To save on prep time, cook the patties on an outdoor grill on medium heat or a Foreman style grill. The cooking time will be greatly reduced; only about 6 to 8 minutes.

Delightful Desserts

Chocolate Chip Banana Nut Torte

Cinnamon Applesauce

Mango-Razz Sorbet

Over the Top Sweet Potato

Succulent Citrus Salad

Vanilla Coconut Milk Ice Cream

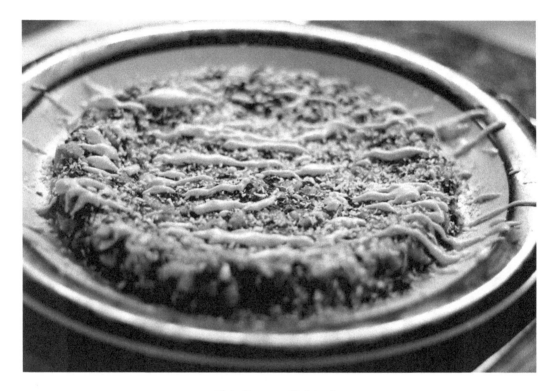

Chip Banana Nut torte

Chocolate Chip Banana Nut Torte

This simple and delicious raw dessert is easy to make and a great choice for dinner parties. For an interesting variation, this recipe can be transformed into a pie crust. All you have to do is press it into a 1/8" layer in a pie dish and freeze overnight. Overall, this dessert contains healthy amounts of folate, potassium, health promoting omega-3 fats from walnuts, blood sugar supporting cinnamon, and the antioxidant power of raw cacao. Prep time: 20 to 25 minutes. Serves 6 to 8.

Ingredients: Organic, local or seasonal
Walnuts – 1¼ cups (whole pieces), pre-soaked, rough chopped
Dates – 3, medjool variety, pitted, pre-soaked, and rough chopped
Raw cacao nibs – ½ cup
Dehydrated whole banana chips* – 2/3 cup, soaked, rough chopped small
Cinnamon – ¼ tsp.
Shredded coconut – sprinkle for garnish
"Banana Coconut Sauce" (see page 77) – drizzle for garnish

*For best consistency of the banana chips, dehydrate them in a food dehydrator at home or pick up bulk-packed, additive-free, dehydrated bananas from a local health food store or online.

Utensils: Chef's knife, cutting board, 3 bowls for soaking, a pair of food service gloves, measuring cup and spoons, mixing bowl, serving platter, pie server, and dehydrator** (optional).

Directions:
- Break up the walnuts as described below, soak them in warm water for about 10 to 15 minutes, and drain.
- Soak the dates in warm water for about 10 minutes (or until soft) and drain. Remove the outer skin of the dates if desired.
- Soak the dried bananas in warm water for 5 minutes or until soft (not too mushy) and drain.
- Rough chop the bananas until smooth and place into a mixing bowl.
- Chop the dates small and place them into the mixing bowl.

Breaking up the walnuts: For a fun way to break up the walnuts before soaking, place them in a sealed storage bag with no air remaining in it. Set it on a solid countertop and gently play the drums on the walnuts with the bottom of your fists. Or, you can swat the bag on the counter until they break into smaller pieces. Of course, be careful not to injure your hands or break the bag while doing so. As the walnuts will breakup easily, it's best to finish up with small walnut pieces instead of walnut crumbs.

- Add in the walnuts, cacao nibs, and sprinkle in the cinnamon.
- With gloves on, mix the ingredients, and pack them together tightly to form a large ball.
- Set out a large dinner plate or serving platter, gently press the ball on it, and use both hands to form it into a circular shape. The finished torte should average between ¼" to ½" high and 7" to 8" in diameter.

Finishing:
- To finish, drizzle on the banana coconut sauce, garnish with shredded coconut, and a few sprinkles of cinnamon.
- Chill it in the freezer until firm (about 1 hour).
- To serve, slice it with a chef's knife and serve with a pie server.

**Dehydrating banana chips:
- Slice a ripe banana into ¼" wide circles, arrange them in a single layer on the dehydrator tray, and set in dehydrator on the dried fruit setting overnight (at least 8 to 10 hours). Seal them in an air-tight container until use.

Cinnamon Applesauce

If you like applesauce, you'll love the super fresh flavor of this recipe and prefer making it over picking up a jar at the store; especially when they are in season. With good amounts of vitamin C, potassium, fibers, and blood sugar supporting cinnamon, this quick and easy prepare dessert is great for anytime. Prep time: 5 to 10 minutes. Makes about 12 to 16 oz.

Ingredients: Organic, local or seasonal
Apples – 4 Granny Smith or mixed variety, cored and rough chopped
Cinnamon – ½ tsp. to 1 tsp.
Lemon – 1 Tbsp., fresh juiced
Stevia powder – 1/8 tsp. or raw local honey - 1 to 2 tsp.

Optional:
Pumpkin spice powder – a dash or two
Maple syrup – 1 tsp.
Cardamom powder – a dash or two

Utensils: Chef's knife, cutting board, measuring cup and spoons, food processor or blender, apple corer/divider, rubber spatula, and a peeler (optional).

Directions:
- Wash and cut the apples as above. Or, if preferred, you may peel the skins* off prior to slicing.
- Blend the apples in the food processor or blender, add in all other ingredients, and blend until very smooth.
- Taste and adjust the seasonings as desired.
- Using a spatula, empty contents into a serving bowl.
- Chill and serve.
- Store and refrigerate in a sealed container and finish within 5 days.

*Although peeling off the apple skins lowers the overall fiber content, the finished texture will be smoother and easier to chew for those with sensitive dental work.

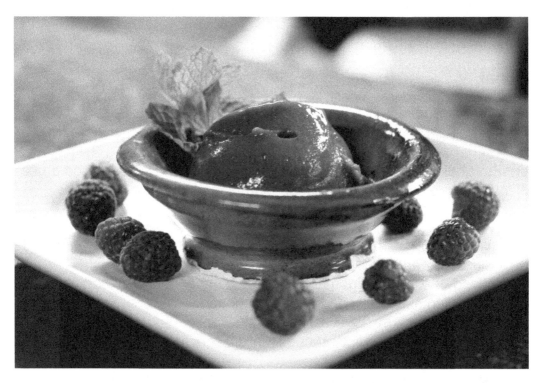

Mango – Razz Sorbet

Mango-Razz Sorbet

With this recipe, you can have fresh, ready-to-go, chill treat in just a few minutes. Most pre-packaged sorbets contain unwanted additives like hi-fructose corn syrup or other added processed sugars. If you are looking to eliminate these from your diet and not lose flavor or nutrition, try this delicious homemade version. A few important things to remember about making this recipe are using the right amount of thickener and having a firm, reliable rubber spatula. Prep time: 5 to 10 minutes. Makes about one pint.

Ingredients: Organic, local or seasonal
Mango – 1 cup (frozen)
Raspberries – 1 cup (frozen)
Apple juice or coconut water – ½ cup (unsweetened variety)
Guar gum – 1/8 tsp. (thickener from the baking section of the market)
Pure stevia or xylitol powder – 1/8 tsp. (if needed)

Optional:
Fruit pectin – 1/8 tsp. (instead of guar gum, found in baking section of supermarket)
Fresh young coconut water – ½ cup

Utensils: Measuring cup and spoons, high speed blender or Vita-mix, rubber spatula, container to freeze sorbet, and ice cream maker*.

Directions:
- In a blender, add apple juice, stevia, thickener, and mix briefly on low speed.
- As you add in all fruit, pulse the blender, and gradually increase the speed until contents are smooth. For best mixing results, occasionally scrape the sides of the blender with a spatula.
- Taste and adjust the thickness with 1 or 2 Tbsps. of apple juice if needed.
- Scoop the contents out with a spatula into a freezer-friendly storage container.
- Allow it to freeze for 2 to 3 hours and serve or enjoy it soft-served right out of the blender.

*If using an ice cream maker, follow the same directions as above then follow the directions given by the ice cream maker manufacturer. This method will help enhance the texture of the finished sorbet.

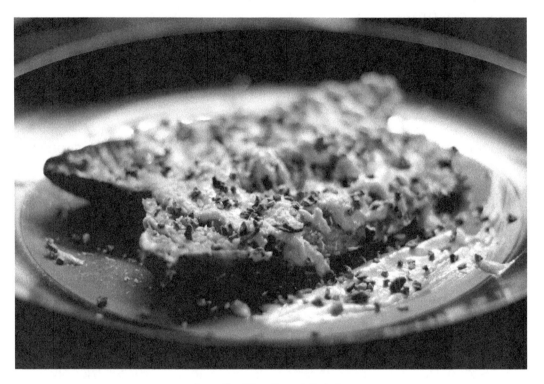

Over the Top Sweet Potato

Over the Top Sweet Potato

With over 13000 IU per serving of vitamin A and so much more to offer in overall nutrition, sweet potatoes make a terrific dessert choice. This recipe was inspired by a happy accident I encountered when some salad toppings fell onto my sweet potato while dining at a restaurant. Luckily, it worked! Prep time: 35 to 40 minutes. Serves 2 to 4.

Ingredients: Organic, local or in season
Sweet potato – 2, medium sized
Extra virgin coconut oil – 1 Tbsp.
Pure maple syrup – brush on skin
Shredded coconut – for garnish
Chopped blanched almonds – for garnish

Banana Coconut sauce:
Coconut milk – 1 cup
Vanilla extract – 2 tsps.
Stevia powder – a pinch or 2 or use pure maple syrup – 1 Tbsp.
Cinnamon – 1/8 tsp.
Flaxseed meal – 2 tsp. (finely ground flaxseeds)
Raw almonds – ½ cup blanched, skins removed
Banana – 1, frozen or fresh

Optional:
Apple – small diced for garnish (Fuji, Braeburn or Honey crisp, etc.)
Cacao nibs – (raw chocolate pieces) sprinkled for garnish

Utensils: Chef's knife, cutting board, baking sheet, pastry brush, blender, measuring cup and teaspoons, saucepan with water for blanching, colander, prep bowl, serving platter.

Directions:
- Preheat the oven to 375.
- Rinse and clean the sweet potatoes.
- On a cutting board, use a fork to poke several holes around the skin of the sweet potato.
- Using a pastry brush spread a thin layer of coconut oil or olive oil on the potato skin and place on a foil lined baking sheet into the oven.

- Bake until soft and a fork goes through the skin easily (about 40 to 45 minutes). Remove from the oven and let cool.

Banana Coconut Sauce:
- While the sweet potatoes are baking, bring water to a boil in a saucepan, add in the almonds, and blanch for about 1 minute.
- Rinse the almonds in cold water and drain.
- Under slow running water, peel off the almond skins, and discard. Save the almonds in a bowl.
- With the blender on low speed, add in coconut milk, vanilla, cinnamon, stevia, flaxseed meal, almonds, banana, and blend until the mixture thickens.
- Blend on high until smooth and creamy.
- Taste and adjust the flavor if needed.

Finishing:
- Over a mixing bowl, brush on a thin layer of maple syrup to cover sweet potato skin.
- Cover the sweet potato skins with sprinkles of the shredded coconut.
- Using a chef's knife, slice the potato down the center (long ways) to open it.
- Gently mash and loosen up the inside of the sweet potato with a small fork.
- Using a spoon, drizzle on the banana coconut sauce over the top of the sweet potato as desired.
- Garnish with a few sprinkles of cinnamon and any of the optional ingredients.
- Chill and serve.

Succulent Citrus Salad

This lightly sweet, juicy and easy-to-prepare salad is terrific for a Sunday brunch, a light breakfast option, and satisfies your hankering for citrus. You'll appreciate this salad even more when you discover some of the nutritional benefits it contains. In addition to its noteworthy water content, this salad provides excellent sources of vitamin A, vitamin C and bioflavinoids, folate, potassium, healthy omega-5 fats, fiber, and many phytonutrients. Prep time: 20 minutes. Serves 2 to 4.

Ingredients: Organic, local or seasonal

Grapefruit - 1 ruby red or pink, peeled and quartered
Blood oranges – 2, peeled and quartered
Mandarin oranges or clementines – 2, peeled, and separated into wedges
Minneola tangelos – 1, peeled and quartered
Pomegranate seeds (arils) – ½ cup, fresh or pre-packaged variety
Cinnamon – ¼ tsp.

Optional:

Mint leaves – 2 or 3, chiffonade (sliced into thin ribbon-like strips) for garnish
Ground flaxseed or chia seed – ½ tsp., for garnish

Utensils: Chef's knife or serrated knife, cutting board, serving bowl and measuring spoons, measuring cup, and compost bin.

Directions:

- Cut and prepare the fruit as above. While removing the peels, try to keep some of the white rind attached to the fruit. There's some beneficial fibers contained in it.
- To finish the fruit, lay the quartered slices on their side, and cut across them 3 to 4 times to form bite sized, even-sized triangles.
- Place all in a large mixing bowl.
- Add in the pomegranate seeds, sprinkle on the cinnamon, flax or chia, and mix with a large spoon.
- Garnish with a few sprinkles of fresh chopped mint leaves and serve chilled.
- Refrigerate leftovers in a sealed container and finish within 3 to 4 days.

Vanilla Coconut Milk Ice Cream

If there's one frozen dessert you can enjoy virtually guilt–free, it's this one. Coconut milk is made from cold-pressing the liquid from the white flesh on the inside of the young coconut. Although it contains saturated fats, these are used more readily by the body for energy, and more immune supporting than processed dairy sources. It also makes an excellent, creamy, dairy-free substitute for making the world's favorite dessert. It's easy to prepare and takes about 20 to 30 minutes in a conventional ice cream maker and comparable in taste, texture, and satiety to regular ice cream. Makes about 1 quart.

Ingredients: Organic, local or seasonal
Coconut milk – 2, 14 oz. cans (chill before preparing recipe)
Pure vanilla extract – 1 tsp.
Pure stevia powder – 1/8 tsp.
Raw agave nectar – 1 Tbsp.
Guar gum – ½ tsp., (thickener, found in baking aisle)
Sea salt – 1/8 tsp.

Optional:
Vanilla beans* – 2, opened and scooped or use a raw, ground pre-packed variety from the raw food section of health food store – ¼ tsp. (easier to work with)
Cacao nibs – ½ cup, (raw chocolate pieces)
For chocolate flavor, add in raw chocolate powder - 3 to 4 Tbsps.

Utensils: Paring knife, cutting board, large mixing bowl, measuring spoons, stand mixer or hand mixer, rubber spatula, can opener, ice cream maker, and a quart-sized freezer container.

Directions:
- In a large mixing bowl, pour in contents of coconut milk and mix well with a hand mixer or stand mixer for about 30 seconds. This helps if there is any separation that occurs in the cans.
- Add in vanilla extract, vanilla bean specks*, stevia, agave, sea salt, guar gum**, and blend well with the mixer.
- Taste and adjust the sweetness, if needed.

Finishing:
- Using a spatula empty the contents into the ice cream maker and follow the manufacturer's specifications to finish.
- Using a spatula, empty the contents into a freezer safe container, freeze for 2 to 3 hours, or simply enjoy it soft serve style.

*To open the vanilla bean, use a paring knife to cut off the tips and carefully slice it down the middle to open. Using the tip of the paring knife or a small spoon, gently scoop out the tiny bean specks.

**Warning: Guar gum is a potent, natural thickener. Keep in mind that a little less is better than too much. Experience with this has taught me that a thick and chewy texture is much less desirable than a smooth and creamy finish.

Part IV
Tables and Resources

Table: pH scale of alkaline and acid forming foods

Healthy Alkaline Foods Eat lots of them	Moderately Acidic Foods Consume in moderation	Acidic Foods Avoid or decrease portion size
Vegetables Alfalfa Grass +29.3 Asparagus +1.3 Barley Grass +28.1 Brussels Sprouts +0.5 Cabbage Lettuce, Fresh +14.1 Cauliflower +3.1 Cayenne Pepper +18.8 Celery +13.3 Chives +8.3 Cucumber, Fresh +31.5 Dandelion +22.7 Endive, Fresh +14.5 French Cut Green Beans +11.2 Garlic +13.2 Green Cabbage Dec. Harvest +4.0 Green Cabbage, March Harvest +2.0 Kamut Grass +27.6 Lamb's Lettuce +4.8 Leeks (Bulbs) +7.2 Lettuce +2.2 Onion +3.0 Peas, Fresh +5.1 Peas, Ripe +0.5 Red Cabbage +6.3 Rhubarb Stalks +6.3 Savoy Cabbage +4.5 Sorrel +11.5 Soy Sprouts +29.5 Spinach (Other Than March) +13.1 Spinach, March Harvest +8.0 Sprouted Chia Seeds +28.5 Sprouted Radish Seeds +28.4 Straw Grass +21.4 Watercress +7.7 Wheat Grass +33.8 White Cabbage +3.3	**Fruits** Apricot -9.5 Banana, Ripe -10.1 Banana, Unripe +4.8 Black Currant -6.1 Blueberry -5.3 Cantaloupe -2.5 Cherry, Sour +3.5 Cherry, Sweet -3.6 Coconut, Fresh +0.5 Cranberry -7.0 Currant -8.2 Date -4.7 Fig Juice Powder -2.4 Gooseberry, Ripe -7.7 Grape, Ripe -7.6 Grapefruit -1.7 Italian Plum -4.9 Mandarin Orange -11.5 Mango -8.7 Orange -9.2 Papaya -9.4 Peach -9.7 Pear -9.9 Pineapple -12.6 Raspberry -5.1 Red Currant -2.4 Rose Hips -15.5 Strawberry -5.4 Tangerine -8.5 Watermelon -1.0 Yellow Plum -4.9 Non-Stored Grains Brown Rice -12.5 Wheat -10.1 **Nuts** Hazelnuts -2.0 Macadamia Nuts -3.2 Walnuts -8.0 **Fish** Fresh Water Fish -11.8	**Meat, Poultry, and Fish** Beef -34.5 Chicken (to -22) -18.0 Eggs (to -22) Liver -3.0 Ocean Fish -20.0 Organ Meats -3.0 Oysters -5.0 Pork -38.0 Veal -35.0 **Milk And Milk Products** Buttermilk +1.3 Cream -3.9 Hard Cheese -18.1 Homogenized Milk -1.0 Quark -17.3 **Bread, Biscuits (Stored Grains/Risen Dough)** Rye Bread -2.5 White Biscuit -6.5 White Bread -10.0 Whole-Grain Bread -4.5 Whole-Meal Bread -6.5 **Nuts** Cashews -9.3 Peanuts -12.8 Pistachios -16.6 **Fats** Butter -3.9 Corn Oil -6.5 Margarine -7.5 **Sweets** Artificial Sweeteners -26.5 Barley Malt Syrup -9.3 Beet Sugar -15.1 Brown Rice Syrup -8.7 Chocolate -24.6 Dried Sugar Cane Juice -18.0 Fructose -9.5

Healthy Alkaline Foods Eat lots of them	Moderately Acidic Foods Consume in moderation	Acidic Foods Avoid or decrease portion size
Vegetables Zucchini +5.7 Root Vegetables Beet +11.3 Carrot +9.5 Horseradish +6.8 Kohlrabi +5.1 Potatoes +2.0 Red Radish +16.7 Rutabaga +3.1 Summer Black Radish +39.4 Turnip +8.0 White Radish (Spring) +3.1 **Fruits** Avocado +15.6 Fresh Lemon +9.9 Limes +8.2 Tomato +13.6 **Non-Stored Organic Grains and Legumes** Buckwheat Groats +0.5 Granulated, Cooked Soy Beans +12.8 Lentils +0.6 Lima Beans +12.0 Soy Flour +2.5 Soy Lecithin (Pure) +38.0 Soy Nuts (soaked Soy Beans, Air Dried) +26.5 Soybeans, Fresh +12.0 Spelt +0.5 Tofu +3.2 White Beans (Navy) +12.1 **Nuts** Almonds +3.6 Brazil Nuts +0.5 **Seeds** Caraway Seeds +2.3 Cumin Seeds +1.1 Fennel Seeds +1.3	**Fats** Coconut Milk -1.5 Sunflower Oil -6.7	**Sweets** Honey -7.6 Malt Sweetener -9.8 Milk Sugar -9.4 Molasses -14.6 Turbinado Sugar -9.5 White Sugar -17.6 **Condiments** Ketchup -12.4 Mayonnaise -12.5 Mustard -19.2 Soy Sauce -36.2 Vinegar -39.4 **Beverages** Beer -26.8 Coffee -25.1 Fruit Juice Sweetened Fruit Juice, Packaged, -8.7 Liquor -38.7 Tea (Black) -27.1 Wine -16.4 **Miscellaneous:** Canned Foods Microwave Foods Processed Foods

Healthy Alkaline Foods Eat lots of them **Seeds** Flax Seeds +1.3 Pumpkin Seeds +5.6 Sesame Seeds +0.5 Sunflower Seeds +5.4 Wheat Kernel +11.4 **Fats (Fresh, Cold-Pressed Oils)** Borage Oil +3.2 Evening Primrose Oil +4.1 Flax Seed Oil +3.5 Marine Lipids +4.7 Olive Oil +1.0		

(Source: "Back to the House of Health" by Shelley Redford Young)

*Each food is assigned a number which mirrors its approximate relative potential of alkalinity (+) or acidity (-) existent in one ounce (28.35g) of food. The higher the (+) number, the better it is for you to eat. The goal to reach is to eat a higher percentage of foods from the (+) category each day. For best results, be sure to drink the proper amount of clean, filtered water in your daily routine. Although this list is not all-inclusive, it will help get you started looking for alkalizing foods while shopping or ordering in a restaurant.

A Few Thoughts About...
Superfoods

Superfoods are the most powerful, nutrient dense, mineral-rich plant foods on earth and are the great gifts given to us by the greatest civilizations that have ever existed. The Chinese civilization gave us goji berries, the Aztecs/Toltecs/Mayans/Olmecs gave us cacao (raw chocolate), and the Egyptians gave us aloe vera. Polynesians gave us noni, the Incan peoples gave us maca, central Africans gave us spirulina, and beekeepers around the world gave us bee pollen, propolis, and royal jelly. Superfoods represent an interesting piece of the nutrition puzzle and supply much more in terms of nutrition density per calorie. They are the best natural sources of clean, pesticide-free, chemical-free, vitamins, minerals, enzymes, antioxidants, co-enzymes, essential fatty acids, healthy fats and oils, essential amino acids, fiber, polysaccharides (glyconutrients or essential sugars), and provide good sources of protein.

According to Wikipedia, "superfood" is a term sometimes used to describe a food with a high phytonutrient content that may confer health benefits as a result. For example, blueberries are often considered a superfood (or superfruit) because they contain significant amounts of antioxidants, anthocyanins, vitamin C, manganese, and dietary fiber. A notable characteristic about this class of foods is they have a higher nutrition density per calorie and contain many scientifically supported health promoting properties.

Superfoods are foods that have medicinal qualities and they offer deep, well-rounded nutritional support. They contain many health promoting properties and immediately go to work to help nourish our brain, bones, muscles, skin, hair, nails, heart, lungs, liver, kidneys, reproductive system, pancreas and, more importantly, our immune system. Over the long-term, superfoods work to correct imbalances, and help to guide us towards a more natural, and original diet. When we consume superfoods, it becomes dramatically easier to achieve our ideal weight, diet, food habits, energize, cleanse and detoxify the body, and satisfy our taste buds and appetite. What more could you ask for? Superfoods promote health and longevity!

The following are considered superfoods: Acai berry, amla berries, aloe vera leaf, bee pollen, bee propolis, blueberries, AFA blue green algae, cacao (raw chocolate), camu camu berries, goji berries, hempseeds, traditional Chinese herbs like Fo-Ti (he shou wu), ginseng, astragalus, or eucommia bark, Incan berries (golden berries), jackfruit, maca root, maqui berries, marine phytoplankton, medicinal mushrooms (reishi, cordyceps, shitake, maitake , chaga, etc.), noni fruit, raw honey, royal jelly, sea vegetables (wakame, nori, kombu, etc.) sprouted vegetables (broccoli, alfalfa, clover, etc.), sprouted seeds (chia, sunflower, pumpkin, etc.) sprouted legumes (chick pea, mung bean, lentil, etc.), sprouted grains (quinoa, buckwheat, wheat berry, etc.) wheat grass, and yacon root, etc.

Other honorable mentions include: almonds, avocados, beans, wild berries, broccoli, cinnamon, leafy greens, tomatoes, garlic, green and white teas, mesquite, onions, pomegranates, quinoa, sweet potatoes, wild salmon, young coconut, etc.

There are several superfoods contained within the recipes of this book. The above list is by no means complete. There are many more being added all the time so I encourage you to learn more about these foods and begin to incorporate the ones that work the best for you.

The following is an excerpt from Dutchovendude.com; a useful website for instant weight and measure conversions. For additional cooking tips, visit this informative page.

Cooking Measurement Conversions

You can't convert cups to pounds. A cup is a measure of volume. A pound is a measure of weight. Would a cup of feathers weigh the same as a cup of gold? No.

Cooking Measurement Abbreviations

Abbreviation	Measurement
Tsp.	Teaspoon
Tbsp.	Tablespoon
Fl.	Fluid
Oz.	Ounce
Pkg.	Package
C	Cup
Pt.	Pint
Qt.	Quart
Gal.	Gallon
Lb.	Pound
Sm.	Small
Lg.	Large

Old-Fashioned Measurements

A pinch, a dash, and a smidgen are a lot like bunch, few, and some; there is no precise measurement. A pinch is what you can pick up between your finger and thumb. Below are some commonly accepted conversions.

Measurement	Equivalents
a Hint	tiny amount (1/2 drop)
a Drop	1/64 teaspoon (1/2 smidgen)
a Smidgen	1/32 teaspoon (1/2 pinch)
a Pinch	1/16 teaspoon (1/2 dash)
a Dash	1/8 teaspoon (1/2 tad)

a Tad	1/4 teaspoon
1/4 stick butter	2 tablespoons
1 stick butter	1/2 cup
juice of a lemon	3 tablespoons
juice of an orange	1/2 cup

Cooking Measurement Equivalents

Measurement	Equivalents						
	tsp.	Tbsp.	fl oz.	Cup	pint	Quart	gallon
1 Tsp.	1	1/3	1/6	1/48			
1 Tbsp.	3	1	1/2	1/16	1/32		
1 Oz.	6	2	1	1/8	1/16		
1 Cup	48	16	8	1	1/2	¼	1/16
1 Pint	96	32	16	2	1	½	1/8
1 Quart	192	64	32	4	2	1	1/4
1 Gallon	768	256	128	16	8	4	1

Selected Internet Resources

Raw Foods and Food Related

Aniphyo.com – Ani Phyo's raw food demonstrations, recipes, links, and information on raw foods.

Annette Larkins – A website featuring a 69-plus year young grandma who looks like a model and teaches about the benefits of raw foods.

Davidwolfe.com – David Wolf's website featuring seminars, workshops on his mission of great nutrition, and sharing information on the health benefits of raw foods with the world.

DrDay - A medical doctor that heals herself with raw foods & juicing.

Gardenofhealth – Portal to excellent sites about raw foods, with articles and more.

Hacres.com - Living foods as related to lifestyle and raw foods.

Learnrawfood.com - An online resource with recipes, menu planning kits, a free monthly newsletter, and books on raw foods.

LivingFoods UK - Provides comprehensive courses on living foods, living foods house party demos, planning for parenthood instruction, phone and personal consultations, a choice selection of living foods equipment newsletter and books on live foods.

Living Light Culinary Arts Institute – A website that teaches the art of raw living food cuisine.

Paulnison.com - Paul Nison's raw food site featuring health and nutrition information, books, DVD's and lectures on the raw food lifestyle.

Rawfoodlife.com – Find out what happens when you eat raw, whole foods, rather than cooked; the science behind raw foods.

Whfoods.org – The world's healthiest foods website started by the George Mateljan Foundation. It's a not-for-profit foundation with no commercial interests or advertising designed to help make a healthier you and a healthier world. It features detailed nutrition information, scientific studies on foods, recipes, videos and many aspects of improving diet and lifestyle.

Pets and Raw Foods

Raw Food for your Animals - Learn about feeding domestic animals in the raw.

Sojourner Farms Homepage - Raw foods for pets in minutes.

Step by Step Pets and Raw Foods - How to prepare raw foods for pets.

Health and Nutrition Products and Resources

Garynull.com – Dr. Gary Null's online store featuring original products, supplements and DVD's.

Iherb.com – An online store to find many nutritional and personal care products at reasonable prices, a useful library of information on supplements and herbs, and many related links.

Mercola.com – Dr. Joesph Mercola's online store containing all-original products, DVD's, etc.

Multipure.com – Water filtration systems for home and business, information on water quality and EPA standards, solid carbon block and reverse osmosis filters; in business for over 40 years.

Myvega.com – Sequel Naturals website for health and nutrition information resources, online store, whole food, plant-based products for meeting daily nutritional needs; based in Port Coquitlam, BC.

Phmiracleliving.com – Dr. Robert & Shelley Young's online store featuring many products to support a healthy pH, health retreats, recipe books and DVD's etc. on living the alkalarian lifestyle.

Sunfood.com – Online market for raw foods, herbs, supplements, recipes and nutrition information.

Sproutliving.com – An organic, raw foods company started by Alex and Mark Malinsky that offers some of the most nutritionally dense food products available on the market.

The company philosophy promotes the following ideas:
   A. Product innovation – the search for superior ingredients that will fill your body with energy, power, and tranquility.
   B. Sharing knowledge – personal truth seeking and insight gathered during research and product development, and sharing these ideas with the community.
   C. Green life – supporting and advocating lifestyles that limit the footprint on our irreplaceable earth.

Swansonvitamins.com – Online store with an excellent selection of supplements, herbs and spices, homeopathic remedies, foods, etc., at affordable prices.

TheRawfoodWorld.com - Shop online for all your raw foods at the Raw World.

Vegetarianusa.com – Great resource for finding health food stores and restaurants for eating healthy while traveling around the U.S.

Websites for Information on Health and Healing

Alkalize For Health - Learn their 8 step program to fight cancer. Emphasis is on alternative treatments, diet, and lifestyle changes that you can do in the privacy of your own home.

Awesomehealth.com – Internet portal for many important health related topics.

Breathing.com - Learn all about the power of the breath and how to increase it.

Drweil.com – A leading resource for education, information, products, services and philanthropic contributions based on the principles of integrative medicine; headquartered in Phoenix, Arizona.

EWG.org – Environmental Working Group; a non-profit organization using the power of information and science to protect public health and the environment.

Garynull.com – Dr. Gary Null's website providing research on many health, nutrition and healing topics, free audio and video podcasts.

Halls.md - Body Mass Index Calculator - Most raw/living foodists generally have a BMI lower than the average population.

Herbaled.org - An educational resource on the Internet for those who seek credible information on the safe and effective use of herbs to promote optimal health and well-being.

Hippocrates Health Institute – A community that offers a natural path for you to heal your body, health retreats to reconnect with your spirit, and rejuvenate your health in West Palm Beach, Florida.

Mercola.com – Dr. Joesph Mercola's website containing many health and nutrition articles, links, free audio and video presentations, online supplement retail store.

Myockn.com – The Center for Alternative Medicine, integrative medicine, health, healing, rehabilitation and wellness resources, food and nutrition classes, online store featuring customized herbal, supplement, and Homeopathic remedies.

Nutraingredients-usa.com – A daily online news service available as a free-access website that provides daily and weekly newsletters to subscribers regarding breaking news on supplements & nutrition in North America.

PCRM.org - Physicians Committee for Responsible Medicine, an interesting site that promotes vegetarianism, many studies, and reports, a wealth of knowledge.

Phmiracleliving.com – Dr. Robert & Shelley Young's health retreat in Valley Center, CA - information on nutritional therapies and products to support a healthy pH, audio, video podcasts, health blogs, health retreats, recipes, products, and books about the alkalarian lifestyle.

Safe-food.org - Information on genetically engineered foods.

The National Green Pages - A thorough directory of products and services for people and the planet.

Tree of Live Rejuvenation Center - One of the world's largest cross-cultural, vegan live-food health restaurants and retreats located in Patagonia, Arizona and run by Dr. Gabriel Cousens.

Whfoods.org – The world's healthiest foods website started by the George Mateljan Foundation. It's a not-for-profit foundation with no commercial interests or advertising designed to help make a healthier you and a healthier world. It features detailed nutrition information, scientific studies on foods, recipes, videos, and many aspects of improving diet and lifestyle.

Selected Bibliography

Appleton, Nancy. Rethinking Pasteur's Germ Theory: How to Maintain Your Optimal Health. Frog Books; 1st edition (May 23, 2002).

Brazier, Brendan. Thrive Fitness: The Vegan-Based Training Program for Maximum Strength, Health, and Fitness. Da Capo Lifelong Books; 1st edition (December 8, 2009).

Campbell, Colin T., Campbell, Thomas M. Campbell II. The China Study: The Most Comprehensive Study of Nutrition Ever Conducted and the Startling Implications for Diet, Weight Loss and Long-term Health. BenBella Books Inc. (Jun 1, 2006).

Calabrese, Karyn. Soak Your Nuts: 1st edition. Healthy Living Publications (January 31, 2011).

Cousens, Gabriel. Conscious Eating: Second Edition. North Atlantic Books (March 3, 2009).

Cousens, Gabriel. There Is a Cure for Diabetes: The Tree of Life 21-Day+ Program. North Atlantic Books; 1st edition (January 8, 2008).

DeYoung, Eric M. How to Live a Happy, Healthy, Wealthy & Safe Life! The Missing Links in Conventional Medicine. Trafford Publishing. (Jan 26, 2011).

Furman, Joel. Eat to Live: The Revolutionary Formula for Fast and Sustained Weight Loss. Little, Brown and Company (January 4, 2005).

Hume, Ethel D. Bechamp or Pasteur? DLM (November 11, 2006).

Mittleman, Stu. Slow Burn: Burn Fat Faster By Exercising Slower. Harper Paperbacks (July 3, 2001).

Murray, Michael T. and John Pizzorno. The Encyclopedia of Healing Foods. Atria; 1st edition (September 20, 2005).

Onstad, Diane, <u>Whole Foods Companion</u>: <u>A Guide for Adventurous Cooks, Curious Shoppers, and Lovers of Natural Foods</u>. Chelsea Green Publishing; Rev Exp edition (March 30, 2004).

Phyo, Ani. <u>Ani's Raw Food Kitchen</u>: <u>Easy, Living Foods Recipes</u>. Da Capo Press (May 7, 2007).

Pitchford, Paul. <u>Healing with Whole Foods</u>: <u>Asian Traditions and Modern Nutrition</u>. North Atlantic Books; 3rd Rev. Upd. edition (February 28, 2003).

Quillan, Patrick. <u>Beating Cancer with Nutrition</u>, book with CD. Nutrition Times Press; 4th edition (May 20, 2005).

<u>Simply Raw</u>: <u>Reversing Diabetes in 30 Days</u>. Lead Editor, Aaron Butler, Raw for Thirty, llc.
DVD released February 2009.

Wehrenberg, Margaret. <u>The 10 Best-Ever Anxiety Management Techniques</u>: <u>Understanding How Your Brain Makes You Anxious and What You Can Do to Change It</u>. W. W. Norton & Company (August 11, 2008).

Wolfe, David. <u>Superfoods</u>: <u>The Food and Medicine of the Future</u>. North Atlantic Books; 1st edition (April 28, 2009).

Young, Robert O. <u>The pH Miracle</u>: <u>Balance Your Diet, Reclaim Your Health</u>. Wellness Central; Revised edition (July 2, 2010).

Young, Shelley Redford. <u>Back to the House of Health</u> (Vol. 1). Woodland Publishing. 1999.

Young, Shelley Redford. <u>Back to the House of Health (Vol. 2)</u>. Woodland Publishing. 2003.

About Chef Peter

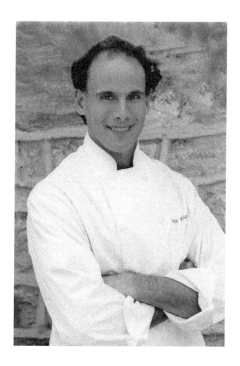

Currently, I live in Louisville, Kentucky working as a private chef consultant and food demonstrator for the Center for Alternative Medicines. I'm also helping to expand a local juice bar business that specializes in offering fresh organic fruit smoothies, superfood drinks, fresh organic juices, bulk herbs, and making delicious and healthy, ready-to-go foods more accessible to the community. In my spare, time I can be found experimenting with new superfood recipes, drumming in a variety of music groups on numerous stages around the world, enjoying the sights and sounds of nature, or jogging from the market with a sack full of produce.